Realize that there is a great wind that blows from heaven and that this wind is Light and Sound. In this stream of Light and Sound, you can dance all the way across the universes. You can turn your consciousness into it, and know that you and the Light are one.

—John Roger—

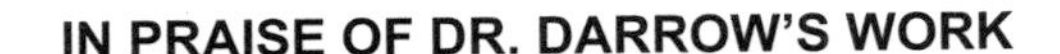

IN PRAISE OF DR. DARROW'S WORK

This book will help change the way pain medicine is practiced. It will teach your doctor how to heal your pain naturally.

Jack Canfield,
Co-author of Chicken Soup for the Soul®

My career as a bodybuilder was destroyed by an injury. Dr. Darrow's unique therapy that he describes in this book literally saved me. I am pain free again and squatting 700 lbs.

Joe DeAngelis,
Mr. Universe, Mr. America

Dr. Darrow's needle feels like an angel dancing on my skin. His treatment gave me my first pain free season in ten years. If you are looking for a doctor who can heal when others fail, read his book.

Johnnie Morton, Jr.,
Pro Football, Kansas City Chiefs

Prolotherapy: Living Pain Free

Marc Darrow, M.D.,J.D.,Q.M.E

Protex Press
Los Angeles, California

Prolotherapy

"Let the Healing Begin"

"Prolotherapy stimulates your body's natural production of collagen and provides relief from chronic pain"

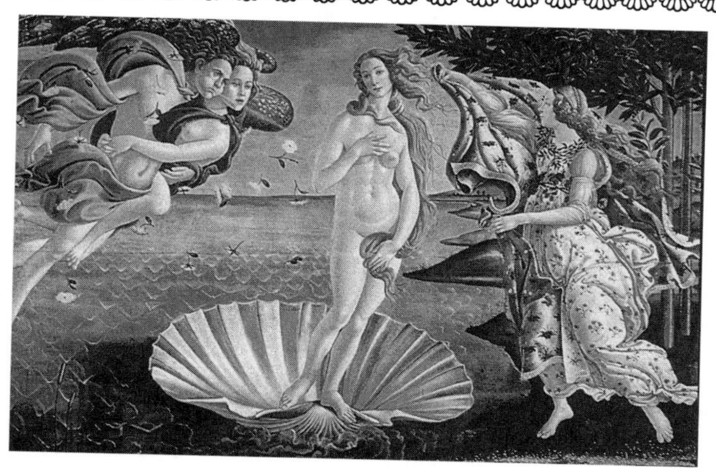

Pearls of Prolotherapy

Pearls are formed when something (a grain of sand, a speck of shell) finds itself inside an oyster and creates irritation.

Since the oyster cannot remove the object, it responds by secreting a nacre, commonly called Mother of Pearl (calcium carbonate), to help soothe the irritation.

The nacre covers the object and continues to coat it until the object ceases to irritate. The resulting incrustation, over several years, produces a pearl, one of nature's most precious jewels.

In this book you will discover how Prolotherapy naturally stimulates the body to rejuvenate itself with the proliferation of new collagen.

Prolotherapy: Living Pain Free
Marc Darrow, M.D., J.D.

Published by Protex Press
11645 Wilshire Blvd, Suite 120
Los Angeles, CA 90025 USA
800-Rehab 10 (1-800-734-2210)
310-231-7000
Fax: 310-231-7227
www.jointrehab.com
lawdoc@marcdarrow.com

ISBN: 0-9714503-2-3

Printed in the United States of America

Dedication (A Practice)

It is difficult if not impossible, with our lives so full of distractions from our inner worlds, to let those we love really know that we love them. This book is dedicated to all of you whom I love. My work is dedicated to you. My life is dedicated to you.

To Michelle, my beautiful wife

To Selma, my loving mother

To Zim, my continuing inspiration from the other side

To Benjy, Jason, Jensen, Jordan, and Britt, my sweet children

To my wonderful partner, Jason Kelberman, and all of our partners in health at Joint Rehab.

Diane Campbell, without her there could have never been this book

Barry Weiner

And that giant of a man who sculpted me from clay, John-Roger.

Disclaimer

This book is designed to provide information about the subject matter covered. It is sold with the understanding that the publisher and authors are not engaged in rendering medical or other professional services. If medical or other expert assistance is required, the services of a competent professional should be sought.

It is not the purpose of this book to reprint all the information that is otherwise available to authors and other creative people, but to complement, amplify and supplement other texts. For more information, see the many references.

Healing the human body is not the responsibility of the practitioner without the total commitment of the patient. It is the patient who must make the commitment and leap of faith to be healed. At the same time, every patient is informed that there are no guarantees.

Every effort has been made to make this book as complete and as accurate as possible. However, there may be mistakes both typographical and in content. Therefore, this text should be used only as a general guide and not the ultimate source of information about healing your pain.

The purpose of this book is to educate and entertain. The author and Protex Publishing shall have neither liability or responsibility to any person or entity with respect to any loss or damage caused or alleged to be caused directly or indirectly by the information contained in this book. In medicine there are no guarantees.

Table of Contents

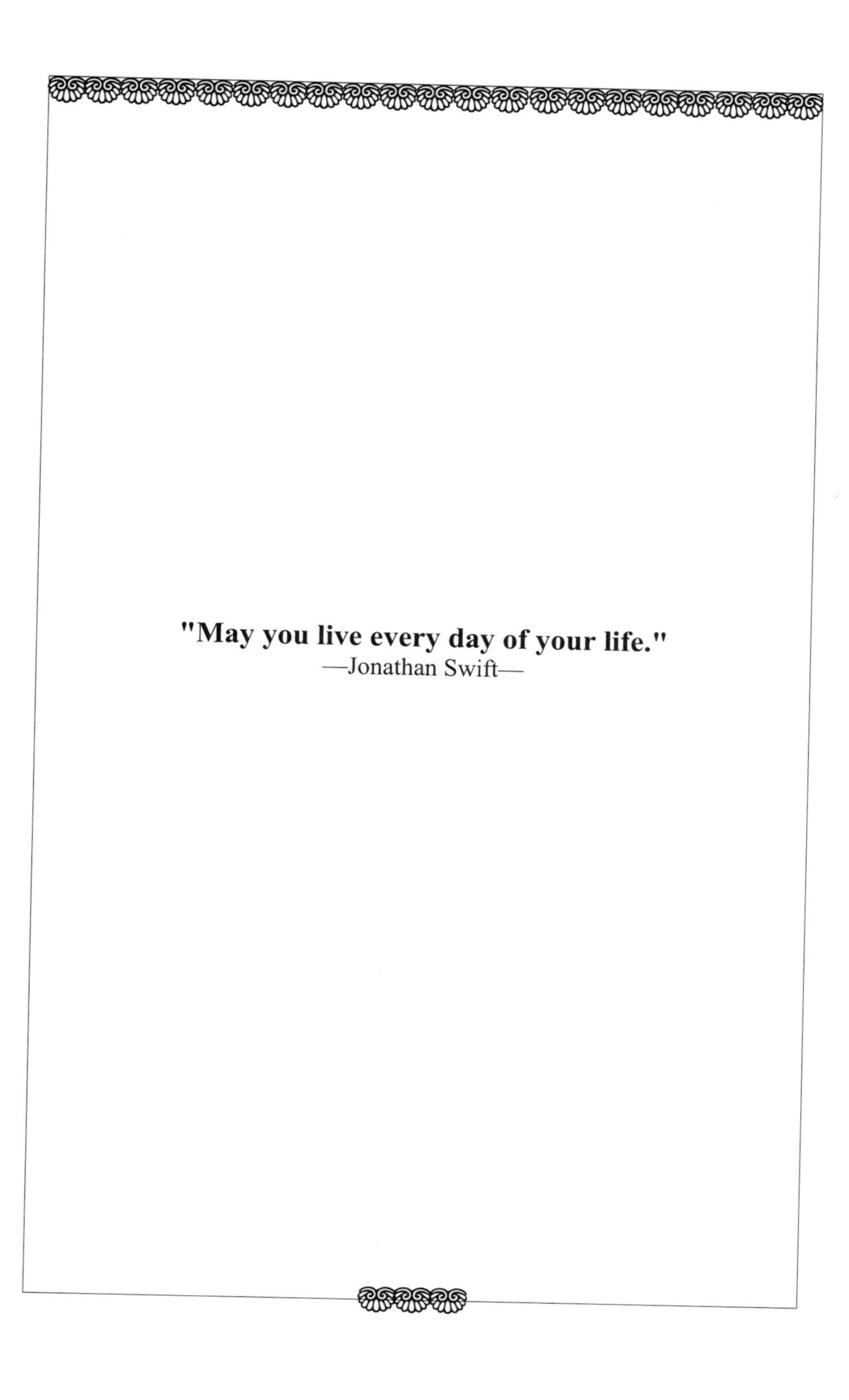

"May you live every day of your life."
—Jonathan Swift—

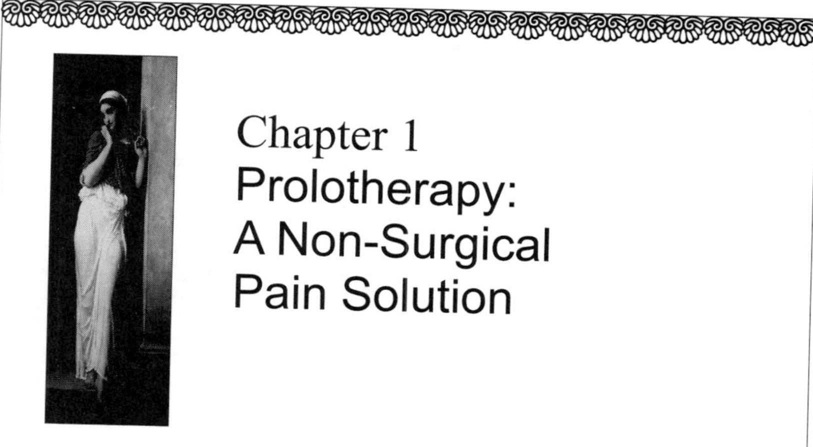

Chapter 1 Prolotherapy: A Non-Surgical Pain Solution

It is said that people who work in Hollywood are always given the best of everything that is new and cutting edge—fashion, technology, and even health care options.

If this were true about health care, then most people who work in the entertainment and fitness industry would not suffer from chronic pain, but they do.

Many of my patients are celebrities and renowned sports figures. They came to our clinic because they were in pain and seeking alternatives to "new and innovative" joint replacement surgeries, "leading edge" arthroscopic surgeries, and an array of drugs and painkillers that did not help them.

What they came to our clinic for was an old-fashioned therapy, first tried and developed nearly 70 years ago. A treatment forgotten for decades because it was "too simple."

I am about to introduce you to a revolutionary therapy that is radically changing the face of orthopedic medicine and the treatment of chronic pain.

It's called Prolotherapy and I personally believe it to be a "miracle," because of the results I have seen achieved by my patients. Their injuries and chronic pain that had plagued them for years, healed with this simple treatment.

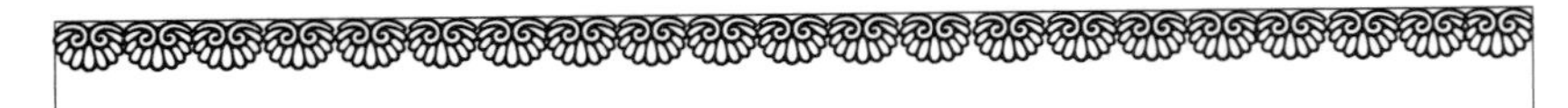

What is Prolotherapy and How Does it Work?

The term "Prolotherapy" is short for "proliferation therapy." Proliferation, of course, means "rapid production." What Prolotherapy rapidly produces is collagen and cartilage.

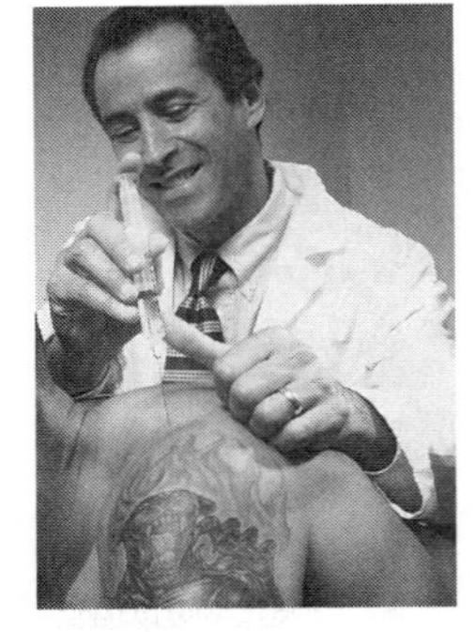

Marc Darrow, M.D., injecting a shoulder

Collagen is a naturally occurring protein in the body that is a necessary element for the formation of new connective tissue—the tissues that hold our skeletal infrastructure together. These tissues include tendons, ligaments, muscle fascia and joint capsular tissue.

Prolotherapy helps make collagen through a series of injections, not of collagen, but of mild chemical or natural (such as dextrose-sugar) irritants, which stimulate the immune system's healing mechanism to produce collagen naturally. The making of new collagen makes for strengthened and restored joints. Restored and strengthened joints makes for permanent pain relief.

The Basis of a Prolotherapy Treatment: The Prolotherapy Doctor's Examination

A Prolotherapy physician will physically examine the patient, being careful to gently press on the suspect area causing pain. When the physician's touch elicits an intense pain spot, known as a ***trigger or tender point***, this is the spot where Prolotherapy is given.

One test you can do at home to determine if you are a candidate for Prolotherapy is to gently press on the area causing pain.

If you can find and put your finger on an exact spot where the pain is coming from, you have found the trigger or tender point, the junction of bone and connective tissue that is injured or weakened.

Prolotherapy is also effective for areas of the body that are painful but not tender to the touch, like the inside of a joint.

The Injections

Unlike the cosmetic use of collagen that requires injecting bovine collagen into the skin to rejuvenate and restore a more youthful appearance, Prolotherapy stimulates your body to produce its own collagen—rejuvenating and rebuilding your body's infrastructure and allowing you a more youthful and pain-free vigor.

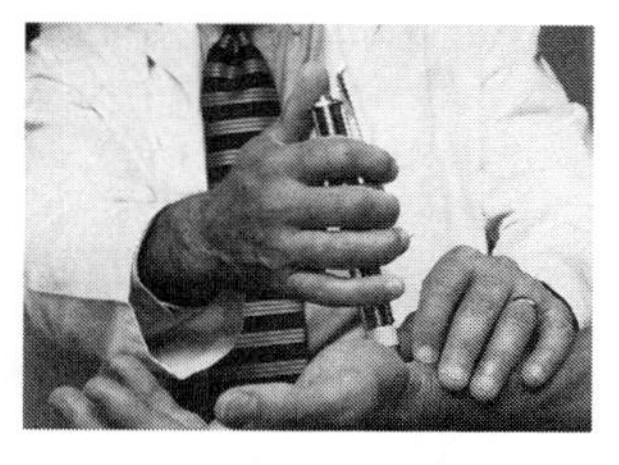

Anesthetic Jet

The ingredients used in Prolotherapy consist of a variety of tested, refined and researched compounds that have been successful in helping alleviate chronic pain.

At our practice at **Joint Rehabilitation and Sports Medical Center, Inc.,** we use a mild dextrose solution in 99% of our cases.

Our practice emphasizes patient comfort. Injections are injections and there are people who hate them, fear them, even get queasy over them.

We make every effort to minimize pain and reduce the stress associated with getting an injection.

Where most Prolotherapists use a long, thick needle, we use a short, very thin needle. This has a significant impact on lessening discomfort. Additionally, we use a "derma-jet" anesthesia spray.

Nearly all the pain associated with an injection occurs at the point where the needle breaks the skin.

A quick spray from the "derma-jet," numbs the skin just before the injection so the patient hardly feels anything.

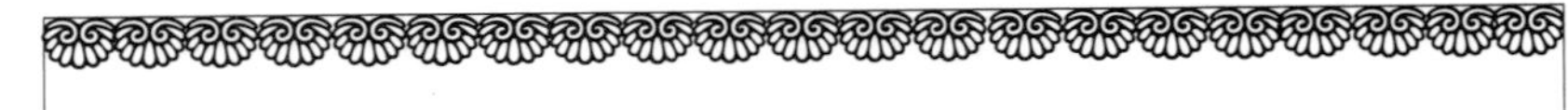

Ingredients

Some Prolotherapists use mild chemical irritants, such as phenol, guaiacol or tannic acid, to trigger the healing process. These substances attach themselves to the walls of the cells wherever they are injected and cause the irritation that stimulates the body's reactive healing process. Others prefer to use chemotactic agents, primarily sodium morrhuate, a fatty acid derived from cod liver oil.

Some Prolotherapists use the dramatic sounding "osmotic shock agents," which are actually simple compounds like dextrose and glycerine. These ingredients are the most commonly used in the arsenal of Prolotherapy and are extremely safe and water-soluble. They are easily excreted from the body after having their initial desired effect. They work by causing cells to lose water, leading to cellular dehydration and then inflammation with its subsequent stimulation of the healing response.

Besides these general differences in the injections, the specific combinations of chemicals and substances used are as varied as the "schools" of Prolotherapy using them.

Some practitioners add co-factors, such as the antioxidant mineral manganese, or a combination of glucosamine sulfate and chondroitin sulfate which is believed to aid in the repair of arthritic joints. Some have preference for other co-factors believed to increase the efficacy of the compounds they are used with.

Although the above methods of Prolotherapy work in different ways—motivating the body to heal itself through a variety of natural responses—the end result is the same: To cure pain by building new tissue and stabilizing the joints.

My Own Story as a Skeptic

I love competition and was once one of the top gymnasts in the state of Illinois. Every sport I participated in, including golf and tennis, was performed with the precision of a gymnast.

...back, neck and joint pain that persisted for years...

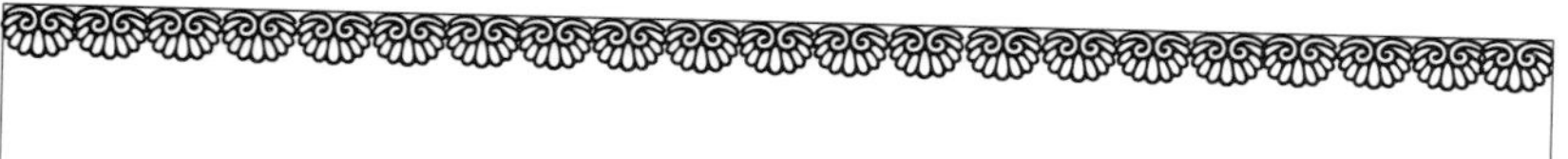

I am still not fulfilled unless I drive a golf ball 300 yards or ace my opponent with a rocket-speed tennis serve. I also lifted a lot of weights, usually until my arms turned black and blue.

By the time I was in my 20's I had racked up my share of injuries. A fall during gymnastics landed me on my tail bone; a high-speed water skiing fall, among many other injuries, left me with back, neck and joint pain that persisted for years.

It wasn't until I severely wrenched my right shoulder while lifting weights that I came to understand how medicine had failed pain sufferers and how Prolotherapy was a "miracle."

After a year of failure with two cortisone injections and physical therapy to rehabilitate my shoulder, a "simple" arthroscopic surgery was performed. I was promised that I would be back to playing sports within three weeks.

After the surgery, in a story that is sadly too familiar, my shoulder became much worse. It blew up like a balloon filled with fluid. Enough so that when I walked, it sloshed.

It took a year after the surgery to return my shoulder to even the baseline pain I had experienced before the surgery. On top of this, chronic neck and back pain, and my right wrist, which had suffered years of abuse from the constant wear and tear of gymnastics, tennis and golf, was bothering me and I had a wicked case of tennis elbow. Pain was my constant companion.

> ***I did sometimes worry that I would be crippled.***

Like many of my patients, I learned to live with pain. After all, I "knew" there would never be a cure.

Being in chronic pain, I did sometimes worry that I would be crippled as the pain extended to different areas of my body. Many of the injuries I suffered in my teens and twenties, which I thought were healed, were revisiting me, one by one.

Then a light turned on. During my fourth year of residency in Physical Medicine and Rehabilitation (PM&R) at UCLA, a PM&R doctor gave a lecture on Prolotherapy.

I immediately liked Andrew Kochan, M.D., because he was more down to earth than other doctors that had taught me. He was a bit radical in his approach, showing how traditional medicine failed those in pain. On this day, his subject was the miracle of Prolotherapy, and he said it helped 80-90% of his patients.

What didn't make sense was why none of us had heard about Prolotherapy.

I was invited to spend time in Andrew's office watching his technique. All the while, it never occurred to me how this therapy would change my life.

Despite my aches and pains, I refused to stop playing sports. During one golf outing a misguided swing caused me enormous pain in my wrist. As I was swinging away, I missed the ball and hit the ground with my club at about 100 miles per hour. My right wrist was forcefully hyper-extended backwards causing me excruciating pain.

The lingering pain was so intense I could barely write. Therapy did not help and the pain would not go away. I had to give up all sports except running. Needless to say, I was miserable.

Dr. Kochan invited me to a medical convention for the American Association of Orthopedic Medicine. During a workshop on Prolotherapy I happened to complain to one of the lecturers that my wrist was probably worse than the one he was describing. He quickly told me that he could fix my wrist with Prolotherapy.

When he explained to me that he would inject my wrist with dextrose and lidocaine, and that this would heal my injury. I had to hide my skepticism.

"Inject me with sugar water? He had to be kidding!"

I was not interested in a shot in my wrist. It hurt enough already! Until that point, although I had watched Prolotherapy and

heard patients rave about it, I never thought I would let anyone inject me. My theory about shots was that it was better to give than to receive. But this doctor was persuasive, and I was desperate. A match made in heaven.

He explained that Prolotherapy worked by causing inflammation at a trigger or tender point where the tissue had been irritated or injured.

The injections stimulate the body's natural healing process. Like the oyster that protects itself from the irritating grain of sand by producing a protective pearl, the human body has its own defense mechanism that promotes healing, it's called inflammation.

"But wait," I thought to myself, "isn't inflammation what causes the pain in the first place? Isn't the reason we take anti-inflammatories to reduce inflammation and pain?"

Later, as a Prolotherapist, I learned that inflammation is your body's siren call. It's nature's way of letting you know that something has gone wrong. The problem with anti-inflammatory pills is that they work by relieving the symptoms, but do nothing to cure the problem. Like winning the battle, but losing the war. While the anti-inflammatory reduces inflammation, it also shuts down the body's natural healing process.

Since I had reached the point where I would try almost anything to fix my wrist and I knew that sugar water would not harm me, I agreed to try Prolotherapy.

How could this happen after months of pain with no improvement?

Then something truly amazing occurred.

I received my first injection and much to my surprise I found the injection to be almost painless. However, my wrist was really stiff for about twenty-four hours afterwards. Although the Prolotherapist told me this was to be to expected, the skeptic in me was working overtime. I thought that not only is this not going to work, but it made my wrist worse.

After about 24 hours, my wrist felt about 50 percent better. How could this happen after months of pain with no improvement? I then went on to inject the wrist myself over the course of the next several weeks.

It was after that when the miraculous occurred. My wrist was almost completely healed. I could hardly believe it myself, but it was true!

I had also cured my tennis elbow and long standing shoulder pain with my own injections. On several occasions, Dr. Kochan, and Dr. Bjorn Eck, an orthopedic surgeon, have injected every vertebrae from my neck to my sacrum. I, thankfully, was back to playing hours of tennis! My sports life was regained.

After my own healing, I started to perform Prolotherapy on any of my patients I could convince to try it.

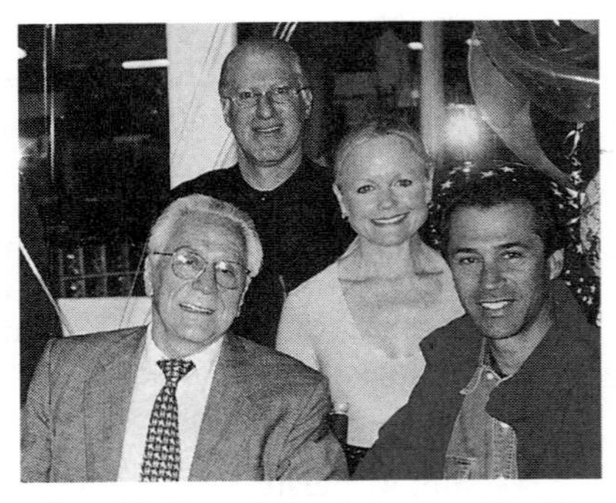

Joe Weider (left sitting) with Dr. Darrow (right), Robert Reiff (Photographer for Weider Publications), and Janet Miller

I Made Believers!

Joe Weider is perhaps one of America's greatest known advocates of health. He publishes numerous magazines about bodybuilding and health, and helped a young Arnold Schwarzenegger and a young Lou Ferrigno become the international fitness icons they are.

I have known Joe for a long time as friend and physician and was grateful he took the time to write about Prolotherapy in my second book, ***The Collagen Revolution***. Here is what Joe wrote.

"I consider myself an evangelist of health. I have spent my life with a single purpose: to bring joy to my fellow man. My focus

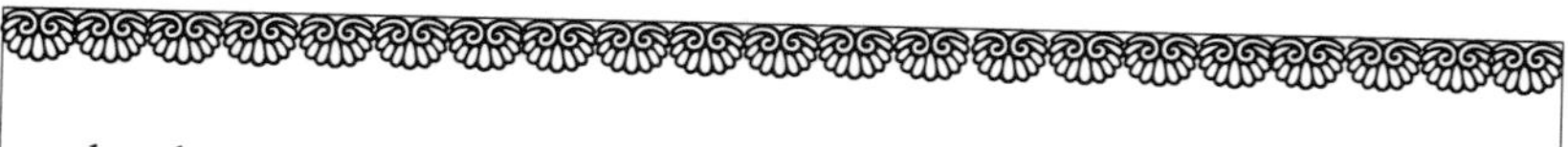

has been to educate the public on the many wonders and paths to excellent health.

Through my own experience, I found that exercise, good diet, and high-minded thinking are all important to maintain a state of well-being. In my process, I have developed among other enterprises, a food supplement company, an exercise equipment line, and seven magazines that focus on health and fitness.

Because of my early success, I have always taken pride in giving talented individuals a stepping-stone to their success.

Part of my good fortune was my referral by my friend and doctor, Leroy Perry, D.C., to a creative healer, Marc Darrow, M.D.

Like many of the current heroes of modern medicine, Marc walks to the beat of a different drummer. His strong spiritual ties have led him to a field that is yet unmapped. He doesn't need devices of the high-tech age to diagnose or treat. He uses his hands and intuition just like his mentors of years past.

Instead of copping out to the surgical quick fix of mainline medicine, Dr. Darrow stimulates the body to naturally heal and rejuvenate itself.

The aphorism, "Physician Heal Thyself" applies in his case since the magical treatment that he administers to his patients was first used on his own body and saved his sports life after years of gymnastics and other sports injuries.

Prolotherapy is the technique that has changed my life and the lives of a multitude of Dr. Darrow's patients. I first learned about it from associates of mine who had experienced miracle pain cures after two or three sessions.

It made no sense to me, and in fact seemed like a fairy tale. I had been treated, without relief, by many of "the best" practitioners, including surgeons and podiatrists, for chronic foot and toe pain. They told me the ligaments in my toes had become stretched from years of athletics such as repetitive toe raises and mountain climbing. Nevertheless, after three to four weeks of Prolotherapy, much of the pain that I had experienced for years, disappeared. As I write this, my foot feels 80% better!

I not only recommend Prolotherapy to those of you who suffer, but I expect you to buy this book for your friends, families, and doctors, and educate them about this therapy. There is new hope for the elimination of your chronic pain."

Joe Weider, Muscle and Fitness Guru

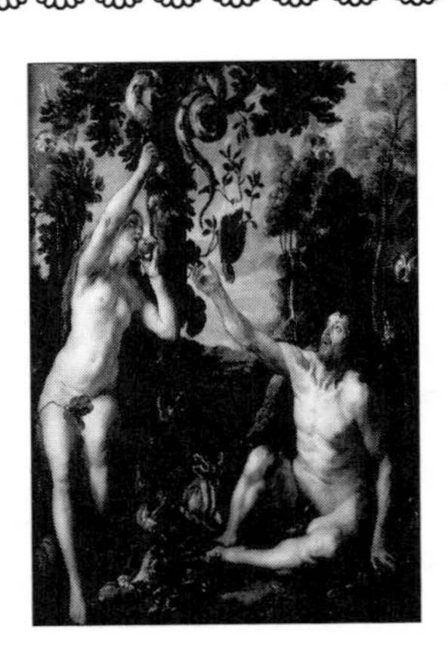

"The wish for healing has ever been the half of health"

—Seneca—

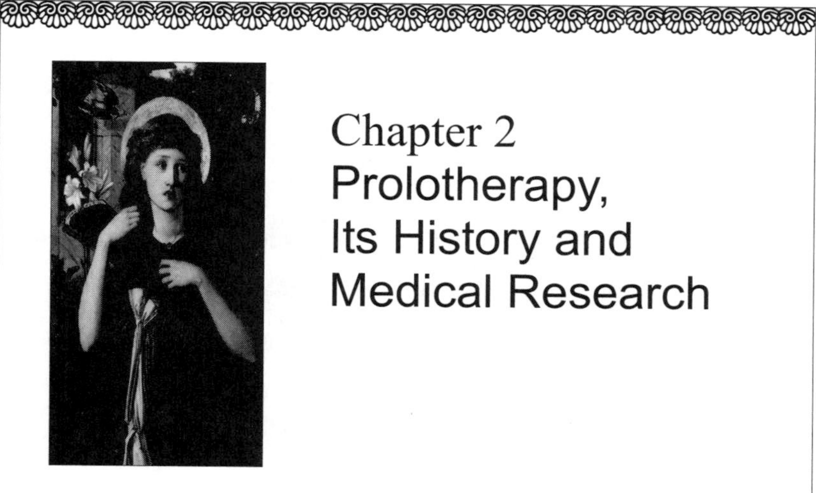

Chapter 2 Prolotherapy, Its History and Medical Research

Prolotherapy is the injection of an irritant solution into the joint, or where the ligaments and tendons attach to the bone. These are the areas where pain is often most intense.

The idea of introducing an irritant into an injured joint is far from new.

Twenty-five centuries ago, Hippocrates, the father of Western medicine, introduced heated metal probes into the dislocated and painful shoulders of javelin throwers. He believed that this would tightened the shoulder capsule by creating tough scar tissue and that the scar tissue would keep the shoulder in place.

In the more modern era, in 1939, Dr. George S. Hackett, a medical doctor working for insurance companies, noticed that car accident victims who suffered from chronic pain, seemed to have chronic pain because of injured or non-healed ligaments and tendons.

Dr. Hackett reasoned that repairing these connective tissues would resolve much of their pain. He introduced an irritating compound to reactivate the body's natural mechanisms to prompt the production or "proliferation" of new collagen tissues. Dr. Hackett coined the term "Prolotherapy" ("prolo" short for

Microphotographs of sections represent the effect of proliferating action on the tissues in the formation of permanent bone and fibrous tissue.

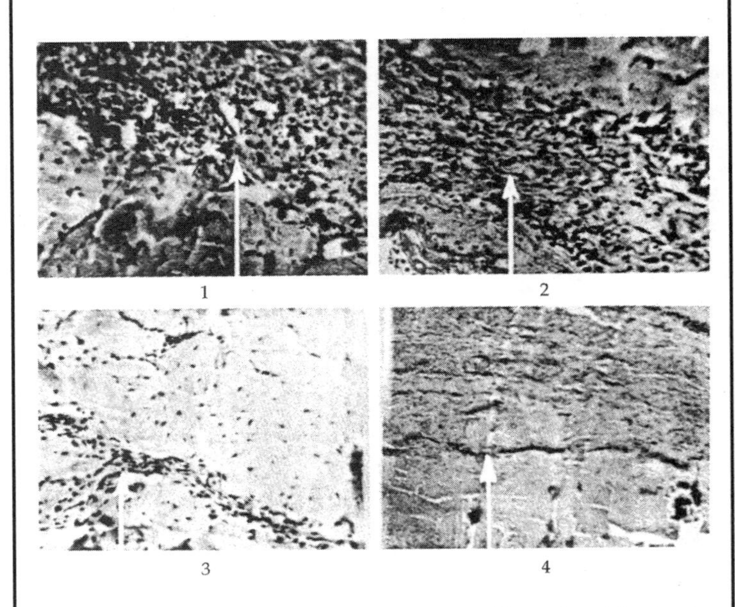

Fig. 29 (1-2-3-4). Microphotographs of sections from rabbit tendons following the injection of the proliferant, Sylnasol (G. D. Searle & Co.), within the fibrous strands. The same technic was used as that which is used clinically.

1) Arrow points to moderate infiltration of lymphocytes 48 hours after injection of proliferating solution. Note absence of necrosis in surrounding tissue.
2) Beginning fibroplastic organization present in adjacent tissues. Arrow points to capillary proliferation with moderate infiltration of lymphocytes. Two weeks after injection.
3) Fibrous tissue now present. Lymphocytic infiltration minimal. One month after injection. Arrow points to few fibroblasts.
4) Fibrosis now present, lymphocytes absent and sheath thickened and fibrosed nine months after initial injection. Arrow points to junction of tendon and its sheath. Nine months after initial injections.

Photographs and x-rays reveal the gross production of permanent bone and fibrous tissue.

"proliferation" therapy) to describe the technique. Dr. Hackett is considered the "father" of modern Prolotherapy because of his extensive research and lectures on the subject, and because he introduced the technique to many other physicians, including Gustav A. Hemwall, M.D.

In 1955, Dr. Hemwall attended a Prolotherapy presentation given by Dr. Hackett at the National Meeting of The American Medical Association. Thoroughly impressed by Dr. Hackett's results in pain management, Dr. Hemwall soon became Prolotherapy's leading practitioner—a role he would continue until his retirement in 1993. Dr. Hemwall's first attempts with Prolotherapy yielded astounding results. Patients who he had treated unsuccessfully for years were suddenly healing and living nearly pain free lives after only a few sessions.

In his career, Dr. Hemwall administered Prolotherapy to over 10,000 patients, one of which was future United States Surgeon General C. Everett Koop, M.D., who, after his own dramatic results with Prolotherapy, offered the treatment to his own patients.

The Medical Rationale for Prolotherapy

Millions of Prolotherapy injections are given each year. But does it work? In chapter one you read my own story. You also read that I was injected with sugar water (dextrose). But, you may ask, isn't sugar water a placebo?

Numerous articles have been published (some of the more important ones are listed below) to determine just that. Is Prolotherapy a placebo? According to the published research, Prolotherapy is not a placebo, Prolotherapy stimulates healing.

Do I need medical validation through scientific review to convince me that Prolotherapy works? You read Joe Weider's story and you will soon read the stories of Sally Kirkland, Jsu Garcia, Amy Gibson, Lamon Brewster and others in the chapters of this book. You also read my own story, not only did Prolotherapy work for my patients and me, it worked like a miracle.

For those who need to see scientific and medical papers before reading further, some of the more regarded papers on Prolotherapy appear on the next page.

Banks, AR. A Rationale for Prolotheapy, J Orthopedic Medicine, 1991;13:55-59.

Hackett GS, Henderson DG. Joint stabilization: An experimental, histologic study with comments on the clinical application in ligament proliferation. Amer J Surg 1955;89:968-973.

Hackett GS. Referred pain and sciatica in diagnosis of low back disabilities, JAMA 1957;63:183-185.

Hauser RA. Punishing the pain. Treating chronic pain with Prolotherapy. Rehab Manag. 1999;12(2):26-28, 30.

Klein R, Dorman T, Johnson C. Proliferant injections for low back pain: histologic changes of injected ligaments and objective measurements of lumbar spinal mobility before and after treatment. J Neurologic and Orthopedic Medicine and Surgery. 1989;10:123-126.

Klein R, Eek B, DeLong B, Mooney V. A randomized double-blind trial of dextrose-glycerine-phenol injections for chronic, low back pain. J Spinal Disord. 1993;6:23-33.

Klein R, Eek B. Prolotherapy: an alternative approach to managing low back pain. J Musculoskeletal Medicine, 1997;May:45-49.

Liu Y, Tipton C, Matthes R, Bedford T, Maynard J, Walmer H. An in situ study of the influence of a sclerosing solution in rabbit medial collateral ligaments and its junction strength. Connect Tissue Res. 1983;11:95-102.

Maynard J, Pedrini V, Pedrini-Mille A, Romanus B, Ohlerking F. Morphological and biochemical effects of sodium morrhuate on tendons. Journal of Orthopedic Research. 1985;3:236-248.

Myers A. Prolotherapy: Treatment of Low Back Pain and Sciatica. The Bulletin of the Hospital for Joint Diseases, April 1961, Vol. 22 No. 1. Initially presented at the 1960 Annual Alumni Meeting Hospital for Joint Diseases.

Ongley M, Dorman T, et al. Ligament instability of knees: a new approach to treatment. Manual Medicine 1988;3:152-154.

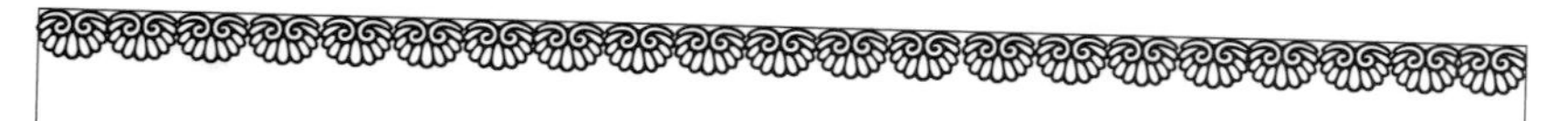

Ongley M, Klein R, Dorman T, Eek B, Hubert L. A new approach to the treatment of chronic low back pain. Lancet 1987;2:143-146.

Reeves KD, Hassanein K. Randomized prospective placebo-controlled double-blind study of prolotherapy for osteoarthritic thumb and finger (DIP, PIP, and trapeziometacarpal) Joints: Evidence of Clinical Efficacy. Altern Complement Med 2000 Aug;6(4):311-20.

Reeves KD, Hassanein K. Randomized prospective double-blind placebo-controlled study of dextrose prolotherapy for knee osteoarthritis with or without ACL laxity. Altern Ther Health Med 2000 Mar;6(2):68-74, 77-80.

Schwartz R. Prolotherapy: A literature review and retrospective study. Journal of Neurology, Orthopedic Medicine, and Surgery. 1991;12:220-223.

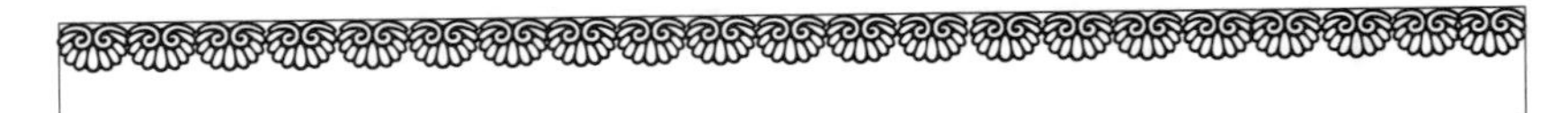

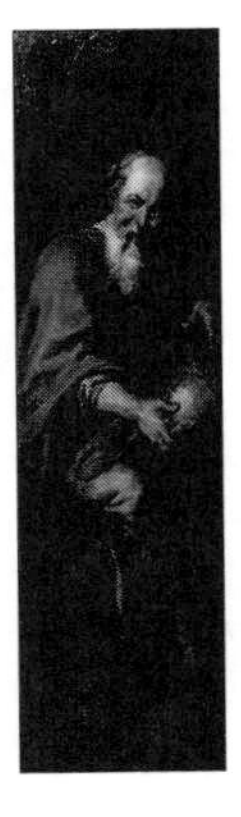

"It is more important to cure people than to make diagnosis"

—August Bier—

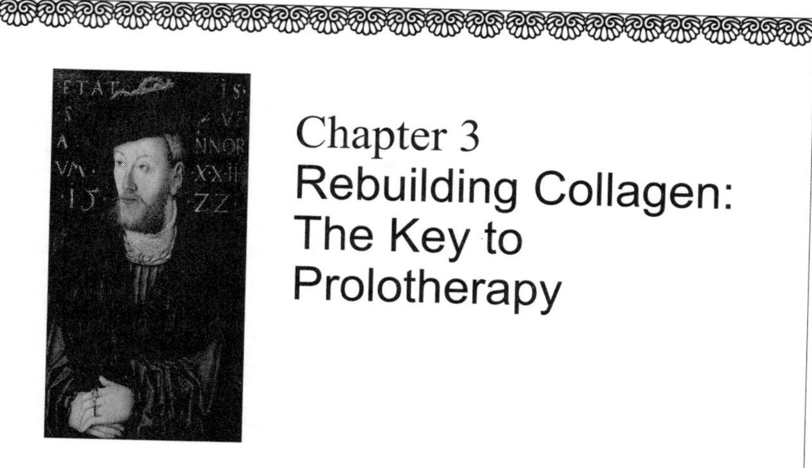

Chapter 3
Rebuilding Collagen: The Key to Prolotherapy

What is Collagen?

Our bones and muscles are held together by the aptly named connective tissue. Connective tissues are ligaments, which connect bone to bone, and tendons, which connect the bones to muscles. It is also the fascia covering muscles and the joint capsule tissue.

Ligaments and tendons are made of collagen. When the ligaments and tendons are injured, the body produces collagen to heal them. The problem with ligaments and tendons is that the body offers them a poor blood supply and, because of it, a poor chance to completely heal.

The poor supply of blood to the ligaments and tendons is very apparent from their white color. Muscles on the other hand are red because they have a very good blood supply. Ligaments and tendons therefore are prone to not heal completely from injury, because their limited blood supply does not offer, among other things, the supplies necessary to rebuild collagen.

Collagen and Degenerative Disease

Most are familiar with collagen because of its cosmetic benefits. Skin is held together by collagen and young skin has plenty of it, making it smooth and wrinkle-free. As we age, the

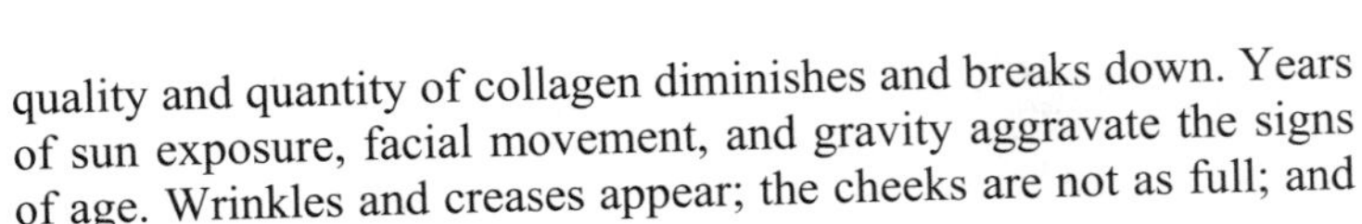

quality and quantity of collagen diminishes and breaks down. Years of sun exposure, facial movement, and gravity aggravate the signs of age. Wrinkles and creases appear; the cheeks are not as full; and the upper lip usually thins out.

Just as the collagen in our face deteriorates, so does the collagen in other parts of our body. This includes the ligaments and tendons in, and around, our joints. Where loss of collagen in our face is signified by wrinkles, in our joints it is signified by pain and a diagnosis of degenerative joint disease or degenerative disc disease.

The key to Prolotherapy is its ability to stimulate the growth of collagen and therefore, the growth of new ligament and tendon tissue. Grow stronger ligaments and tendons and you repair the injury and reverse the degenerative cycle of arthritis and wear and tear disorders.

A Profile of Collagen

Collagen makes up 70-90% of the stuff that holds our bones and joints together and in their proper place. Some older readers may remember that old horses were often sent to the "glue factory." The reason is that boiled collagen is used as glue.

In degenerative disease and aging, collagen, like glue, dries out and loses its ability to stretch. Why this happens more in some individuals than others is speculation at this time. There are many theories including, but not limited to, poor genetic makeup, blood type with its specific dietary requirements, viral or bacterial load, pathological conditions, acidity in the body, and food allergies, to name a few.

But just as collagen can rejuvenate damaged skin to make you look better, collagen can rejuvenate your soft tissues to help eliminate your pain.

Collagen and Joint Injuries

In non-injured ligaments or tendons, collagen fibers are flexible and have some elasticity. Elastic as they are, they are not supposed to stretch very far. Injuries occur when we stretch these

fibers beyond their designed lengths. Injuries also occur when wear and tear through repetitive motion fray and tear at these fibers.

When these tissues are stretched beyond their normal limits, wear out, or tear, pain is perceived.

Inflammation produces pain, which is a sign the body's healing process is occurring. So initially, inflammation occurs as the body tries to heal the damage. Since the tendons and ligaments have a poor and limited blood supply, it is important not to shut down the initial inflammatory response (as you will read in the following chapter on painkillers and anti-inflammatories.) Shutting down the inflammation is equivalent to shutting down the healing cycle and YOU prevent yourself from healing correctly.

In all cases that require Prolotherapy, the ligaments and tendons, whether through the use of anti-inflammatories, or because of a weakened immune system, or because of the severity of the injury, did not heal sufficiently.

When things do not heal correctly, not only is there chronic pain, but now inflammation, initially our friend, also becomes chronic and bothersome.

Injured, loose, or stretched out ligaments are often referred to as ligament relaxation, or ligament laxity. This is what produces the pain and discomfort, especially with movement. Because of the laxity, the joint may move beyond its normal range of motion.

Referred Pain

Pain will not only occur at the site of the injury and loose ligaments, but may also be referred to other parts of the body.

Referred pain is created by ligament laxity around a joint, but is felt at some distance from the injury. These painful points that refer pain elsewhere are called trigger points, and will be dealt with later. Abnormal joint movement also creates many "protective actions" by adjacent tissues. Muscles will contract in spasm in an attempt to pull the joint back to the correct location or stabilize it to protect it from further damage.

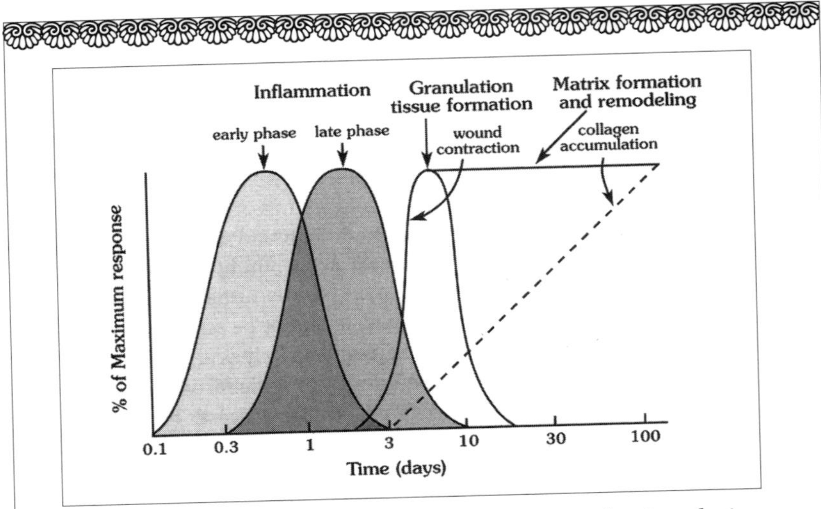

The Inflammatory response with collagen production during the healing of an injury.

When this occurs in the back, orthopedic surgeons will often try to reduce vertebral instability by fusing the vertebrae with bone and/or metal fixation. But there is often an easier and more conservative way to achieve the same stabilization. And this is the outcome of Prolotherapy.

Unfortunately, this is where chronic problems begin, because the conventional medical practice with its emphasis on pain relief, treats the symptom—pain, and not the problem—laxity. A patient will likely be told to take anti-inflammatory drugs, which is often precisely the wrong thing to do because inflammation is the first part in the body's healing process.

Nonsteroidal anti-inflammatories (NSAIDS) and cortisone (an anti-inflammatory steroid) can give immediate relief, but with a risk of creating a long-term injury with chronic pain.

By blocking inflammation, anti-inflammatories never allow complete healing, and instead, aggravate the situation.

Inflammation and the Healing Process

If we allow the inflammation process to run its cycle without interference, we see that inflammation leads to granular tissue formation that results in new collagen tissue being created. The new collagen forms new threads, which attach themselves to the damaged tissue.

New collagen fibers are short, they lose water and shrink, and as they attach themselves to the old ligament, muscle, joint capsule, or tendon, these tissues become more dense. Denser tissue is stronger tissue. This process is much like the scab on a wound or scar that tightens up and shrinks once healing occurs. The difference is that with Prolotherapy, biopsies have shown brand new, beautiful tissue without evidence of scarring. In essence, the tissue is healed, rejuvenated and made stronger than before.

The Science Behind the Regrowth of Collagen with Prolotherapy

As we have noted, the collagen in our bodies, especially in the tissue around and near our joints, is prone to breakdown. We subject our joints to wear and tear through repetitive movement, injury, accident or any other number of reasons. Because the connective tissue around our joints and cartilage have poor blood circulation, conventional treatment maintained that any injury to connective tissue was often irreparable. This was before a study conducted by Y. King Liu.

In a 1983 study of Prolotherapy's effectiveness, Y. King Liu injected five percent sodium morrhuate solution into the medial collateral ligaments of rabbits. He found that after five injections, the ligament mass increased by 44 percent, the thickness by 27 percent, and the strength of the ligament bone junction increased by 28 percent[1].

Liu's study[1] confirmed the results of an earlier study done by George Hackett[2], M.D. In 1955, Dr. Hackett and his colleague Dr. D.G. Henderson, reported on two years experimentation on the effects of the proliferant Sylnasol when injected into rabbit tendons.

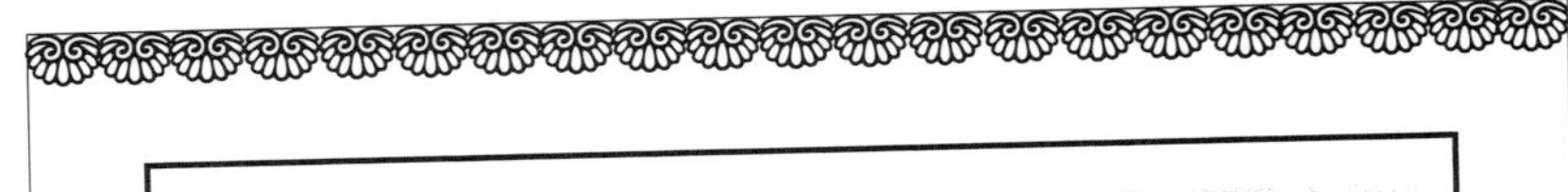

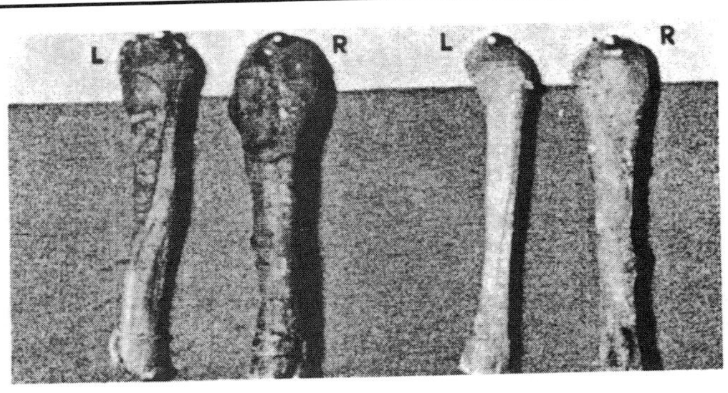

9 months 12 months

Fig. 30. Photograph of rabbit tendons at nine and 12 months after three injections of proliferating solution into the right tendons. Left, controls; right, proliferated. The tendons on the right reveal an increase in diameter of 40 per cent, which is estimated to double the strength of the tendon. The upper portion reveals the attachment of the ligament to the bone which has increased 30 per cent in diameter. The proliferating solution stimulates the production of new fibrous connective tissue cells which become organized into permanent non-elastic fibrous tissue.

In 48 hours, histological tissue examinations revealed an early inflammatory reaction surrounding the nerves and blood vessels with lymphocytic (immune system cells that remove damaged tissue) infiltration throughout the area between the two tendons and between the tendons and its sheath.

Two weeks after the injection, fibrous tissue was present; lymphocytic infiltration had diminished, although some was still present, which showed that the proliferation of new white fibrous tissue was still being stimulated.

One month after injection, fibrous tissue was present, and lymphocytic and fibroblastic (immune system rebuilding cells) activity was greatly diminished. In other words, they finished their jobs and moved on.

As you can see from the illustration above, one year after

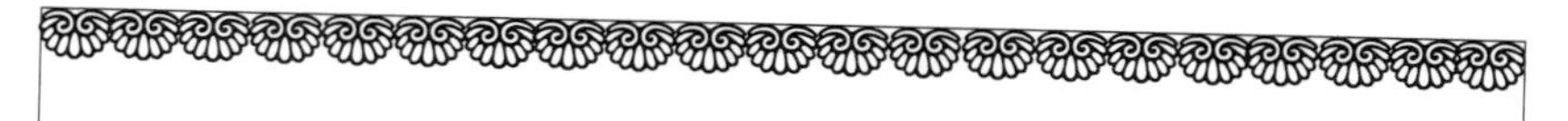

three injections of the proliferant solution, the diameter of the tendons increased dramatically, which was estimated to double the strength of the tendon.

References

1. Liu Y, Tipton C, Matthes R, Bedford T, Maynard J, Walmer H. An in situ study of the influence of a sclerosing solution in rabbit medial collateral ligaments and its junction strength. Connect Tissue Res 1983;11:95-102.

2. Hackett GS, Henderson DG. Joint Stabilization: An experimental, histologic study with comments on the clinical application in ligament proliferation. Amer J Surg 1955;89:968-973.

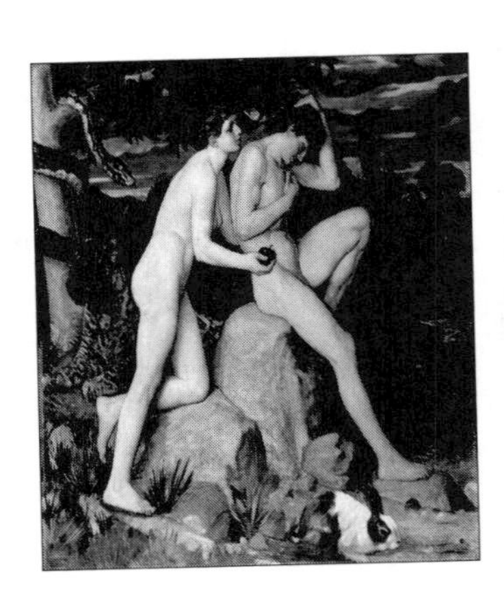

"When you get sick and tired of being tired and sick—you'll change"

—John Roger—

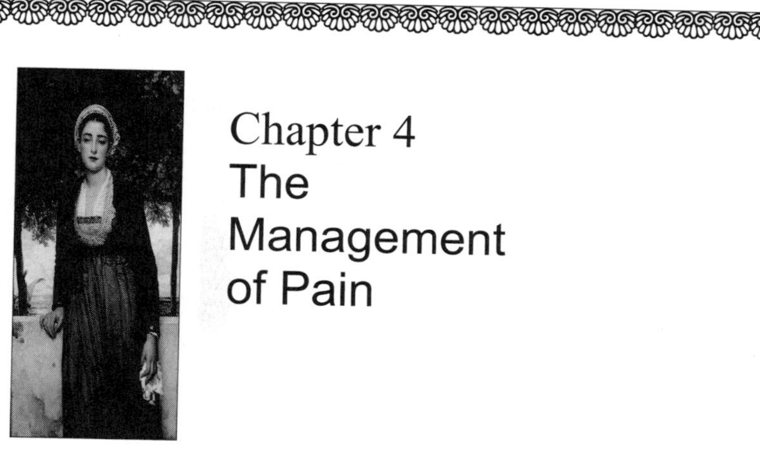

Chapter 4 The Management of Pain

If there were a pill that could rebuild tendons and ligaments through the stimulation of collagen growth, it would be hailed in the medical community as a miracle breakthrough. Unfortunately we haven't reached that stage of medicine yet. I know most of my patients would rather have their Prolotherapy dispensed in pill form.

I also know that almost all my patients would rather have tolerated a few injections of Prolotherapy rather than have a surgical procedure—had they known about Prolotherapy before the surgery.

A familiar expression of gratitude and joy of being pain free after years of chronic pain is, ***"Doc, if I only had known about Prolotherapy years ago."***

The Epidemic of Pain

If you have pain, you are hardly alone.

Eighty-six million Americans have it, it costs about $90 billion dollars annually to try to remedy it, and according to data from the **National Center for Health Statistics**, musculoskeletal system surgeries are the second leading type of surgery performed in the United States annually.

Myofascial pain syndrome is one of the most common disorders seen in chronic pain clinics.

It occurs when damage or injury in the soft connective tissues does not heal properly.

At the site of the injury or damage, "trigger points" develop. Trigger points are hyper-irritable bundles of muscle fiber, ligament, or tendinous soft tissue that produce both local and referred pain when pressed. Tender points are similar, but do not refer pain.

Trigger or tender points have been associated with all sorts of soft tissue injuries that result in patient complaints of headache, neck pain, low back pain, knee pain and various other musculoskeletal disorders. Patients with active trigger points typically complain of pain—which may be characterized as either sharp or dull, localized muscle spasm or weakness, as well as generalized fatigue and malaise.

Painkillers and NSAIDs

The body's natural healing response is inflammation. Inflammation is the trigger for the cascade of events that follow in wound and injury repair. In my opinion, the moment inflammation became the enemy of healing, is the moment chronic pain started becoming a billion-dollar business for drug companies.

When Ibuprofen was introduced in 1974, it was heralded as one of the great steps in the management of pain. By 1976, two years after its introduction, 1.7 billion tablets had been produced.

Today, over 100 million prescriptions for pain relievers are written annually and 15 tons of aspirin are consumed each day. Yet chronic pain persists. Why?

Because these drugs only mask the problem of pain and do not attempt to cure it.

Furthermore, these drugs come with their own risks of addiction and unpleasant side effects.

Anti-inflammatory drugs like aspirin and ibuprofen taken for pain-related problems account for one-third of all the side effects reported by the Food and Drug Administration.

More than 100,000 people are hospitalized each year for gastrointestinal complications resulting from the use of anti-inflammatory medicines, and over 16,000 deaths can be attributed to these complications.

If you suffer from myofascial pain, joint pain, arthritis, sprained or strained ligaments, almost any kind of pain, most likely your doctor will prescribe one of the non-steroidal anti-inflammatory drugs, or NSAIDs listed below. These drugs will reduce the inflammation, which in the short-term reduces the pain. However, in the long-term they set you up for more pain and long-term chronic injury and worse.

In our practice, many alarmed patients have had to stop the use of NSAIDs because of stomach discomfort, nausea, and dizziness.

Newsweek covered this topic in their September 3, 2001 issue. In talking about of the side effects of anti-arthritis drugs, the article relays fears about two NSAIDs that were heavily advertised and marketed directly to consumers. These caused concern when "a leading cardiologist reported that the two drugs could pose a small but disturbing additional risk of heart attack."

The ***Newsweek*** article goes on to note that "for drug companies, arthritis has been a boon: a non-fatal, incurable disease that may require patients to take pain-relief medication every day for

If all this was not enough, beyond the potential side effects NSAIDs can cause, they may also contribute to more pain in the future!

Studies have shown that those who used a strong NSAID, had more cartilage destruction of the hip than those who didn't use NSAID.

Although NSAIDs block inflammation, they apparently interfere with cartilage biosynthesisis, or can have negative effects by some unknown mechanism.

A list of NSAIDs*
(Non-steroidal anti-inflammatory drugs)

Aspirin
Ibuprofen (Advil, Motrin)
Carprofen (Rimadyl)
Celecoxib (Celebrex a Cox.2 inhibitor)
Choline Magnesium Trisalicylate (Trilisate)
Choline Salicylate (Anthropan)
Diclofenac (Voltaren)
Diflunisal (Dolobid)
Etodolac (Lodine)
Fenoprofen calcium (Nalfon)
Indomethacin (Indocin)
Ketoprofen (Orudis)
Ketorolac tromethamine (Toradol)
Magnesium salicylate (Doans, Magan, Mobidin)
Meclofenamate sodium (Meclomen)
Mefenamic acid (Ponstel)
Naproxen (Naprosyn)
Naproxen sodium (Aleve, Anaprox)
Piroxicam (Feldene)
Sodium salicylate
Tolmetin (Tolectin)
Vioxx
Bextra

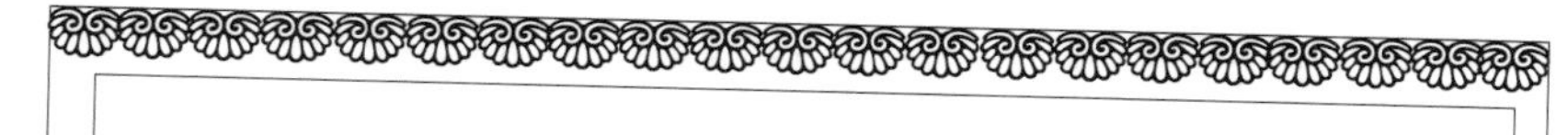

*Potential Side Effects of Aspirin and Some NSAID's**

Gastritis, esophagitis, bleeding ulcers
Renal (kidney) insufficiency
Liver abnormalities
Fluid retention
Platelet inhibition (and therefore possible prolonged bleeding)
Tinnitus (ringing in the ears)
Exacerbation of asthma

Corticosteroids

Cortisone & Prednisone (most commonly used steroids)

Potential Complications of Steroid Use*
Growth retardation in children
Cataracts
Osteoporosis
Aseptic necrosis of the femoral head
Proximal myopathy
Delayed wound healing
Decreased resistance to bacterial and yeast infections
Buffalo hump
Skin striae
Mood disturbances
Psychosis
Adrenal suppression
Cushing's syndrome
Increased blood pressure
Glucose intolerance
Restlessness, nervousness, insomnia
Increased appetite
Weight gain
Hirsutism (increased body hair)
Gastrointestinal bleeding

decades. Since their introduction in 1999—(these drugs) have captured more than 60% of the $6.6 billion arthritis drug market—a figure that doesn't even include products like acetaminophen, which are used to treat other conditions as well."

***These medications are not as benign as many people, including doctors, think and should not be taken long-term for the management of chronic pain.**

NEVER SIMULTANEOUSLY TAKE TWO OR MORE OF THESE MEDICATIONS WITHOUT THE ADVICE OF YOUR DOCTOR!!!!

Why You May Win the Battle, BUT Lose the War

Understandably, people do not like to feel pain and would like to prevent it at all costs. They want immediate relief and getting rid of the inflammation often provides that relief.

The basic truth is that immediate relief does not equal long-lasting relief. Interfering with the body's healing process by stopping inflammation to reduce pain causes long-term suffering down the road.

Inflammation does cause pain, but, pain can be your friend. It is the body's siren alerting you that you have injured yourself. Getting rid of inflammation with NSAIDs provides some immediate relief from pain. It sets you up to win the battle, but lose the war.

By stopping inflammation we shut down the body's natural healing which inhibits the growth of new tissue.

Inflammation, and the accompanying pain, are actually your allies in healing.

"Hey, that sounds like me."

Partners Against Pain, an educational program sponsored by Purdue Pharma, commissioned a survey whose results were published on November 15, 2000 and released to the national news media. Some of the survey highlights are below.

I am willing to bet you will read the following and say, ***"Hey, that sounds like me."***

Q. ***Are you so dissatisfied with the effectiveness of your prescription and over-the-counter pain medications that you are willing to try new treatments?***

If you said yes, you would be part of the seventy-eight percent of the people surveyed who were—and were—willing to try something new.

Q. ***Would you gladly pay more for a pain treatment if you knew it would work for you?***

If you said yes, you joined 43% of the people surveyed.

Q. ***Do you think your over-the-counter pain medication is completely effective or very effective?***

If you said no, you would join two out of the three people surveyed who found their medications NOT to be effective.

Q. ***Have you experienced pain for over five years?***

If you said yes, you joined 62% of those surveyed.

Q. ***Are you satisfied with the way your doctor is managing your pain?***

If you said no, you joined 62% of those surveyed. Additionally those with a negative view of their physician's pain management program said they were most dissatisfied with the treatments the physician offered and the belief that their doctor was not "doing as much to heal me as he/she could."

Q. ***Have you seen at least three physicians for your pain?***

If you have, you are an average pain sufferer.

Q. ***Have you taken about four prescriptions for your pain?***

If you have, you are about an average pain sufferer who takes 3.7 prescriptions for pain.

Q. ***Would you be willing to travel more than 51 miles for pain relief from a medical clinic?***

If you said yes, you would be the one in five who would do so.

In my practice, many of our patients have seen up to a dozen or more practitioners. Many of these patients travel to our clinic from around the country seeking Prolotherapy and our other services.

Prolotherapy and Long-Lasting Healing Inflammation Is Good

In the preceding pages you read about the drug industry's absolute desire to eradicate inflammation. Now I am going to tell you about Prolotherapy's use of inflammation in its most beneficial form.

During inflammation the blood vessels in the area of injury expand and leak, causing the swelling that is experienced.

This expansion enables more blood to flow into the injured area. However, the pressure irritates sensory nerves, and produces the pain that you feel.

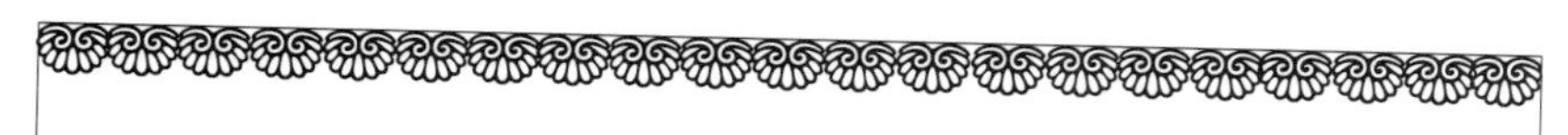

In the fluid are white blood cells and other immune cells, such as macrophages, whose job it is to destroy and remove bacteria, foreign bodies, and dead tissue.

Once finished, these cells are replaced by fibroblasts, which are cells whose job it is to repair the damaged area by laying down new collagen to strengthen connective tissues.

Once new collagen formation occurs, pain is greatly reduced, if not entirely eliminated. The damaged tissue is rejuvenated and often stronger than before.

If it's instant gratification you want, anti-inflammatories are an option, but only short-term. They are likely to do more harm than good, and can lock you into a cycle of chronic pain.

So most doctors, unaware of Prolotherapy's abilities, go ahead and treat their chronic pain patients with their number one tool—sedation!

It is unfortunate more physicians do not utilize Prolotherapy. It is even more unfortunate that very few physicians have even heard of Prolotherapy.

Without big drug money behind it to create major scientific studies, Prolotherapy may remain a treatment off the beaten medical path. It is mainly the testimonials of healed patients that inform the medical profession of the efficacy of Prolotherapy.

Why won't drug money sponsor Prolotherapy research?

Because you can't patent sugar water or any of the other natural ingredients in the injections. No patent, no big money, no research, no advertising.

So most doctors, unaware of Prolotherapy's abilities, go ahead and treat their chronic pain patients with their number one tool—sedation.

I am against the chronic, daily use of narcotics. Patients become tolerant to them and live in a depressed state of consciousness. Patients on narcotic prescriptions give up on life and are harder to help heal.

At our clinic, we handle pain with many modalities that allow our patients to be weaned off their painkillers.

There have been many studies and theories presented as to how to alleviate the pre-conceived or conceived notion of pain. If this can be accomplished, many chronic pain sufferers could see a drastic reduction in their chronic pain and need for drugs.

Many researchers believe that the key to overcoming chronic pain may be locked in the brain. If one can manage stress, pain management is facilitated.

This idea is based on the work of psychologist Ronald Melzack and anatomist Patrick Wall. Melzack and Wall first proposed their theory in 1965 that nerve impulses (pain waves) had to pass through a "cellular gate" to get to the brain's pain center and that is was possible to close this gate and prevent the pain impulse from reaching the brain and causing the pain sensation.

Many researchers agreed that psychological factors (including stress) left this gate open and pain to be felt. Reducing stress, fears, mood, and emotion, would help keep this gate closed.

Pain, a Tough Friend

Pain is a friend, smart and vigilant, ready to point with relative precision at any problem that indicates something is not right with our bodies. We need to listen to it.

After a long period of "mourning" because I could not play golf, secondary to an elbow injury from playing too much golf, I was told in a dream that the injury was in essence a gift. At first I didn't understand. Then I got it, I was out of sync with my work and family because I was escaping to the golf course at every

possible moment. I was secretly distraught because I was not tending adequately to my personal and family responsibilities.

When I realized that the injury gave me more time to be responsible, I was actually much happier overall, it made me think about the positives of pain. This is not always easy to do in dire straits. At the same time we must use everything to our advantage, and it does no good to feel sorry for yourself. Believe me, I've tried without success. I look at every person's pain as a message. I'm certainly not the judge of what the message is, but I present the options to my patients that all messages in one way or another force us to look inside. Pain is possibly the greatest messenger.

The Pain Signal

The pain signal is our body's first line of defense. Without such warning, a person with a broken leg might attempt to walk and permanently ruin the leg.

Pains might be sharp, dull, aching, burning, lingering, or imaginary; or possess countless other attributes or combinations thereof. But whether real or imagined, pain is always a clue to a genuine problem of some sort, whether small or serious, physical or psychological, and often it is a combination of the two.

Prolotherapy allows us to show a patient a tool that when used, for the proper conditions, can bring them their long sought after relief from pain. Show a patient this tool and start closing some pain gates.

References

Agrawal NM. Epidemiology and prevention of non-steroidal anti-inflammatory drug effects in the gastrointestinal tract. British Journal of Rheumatology 1995; 34:5-10.

Bartle WR, Gupta AK, Lazor J. Nonsteroidal anti-inflammatory drugs and gastrointestinal bleeding: A case control study. Arch Intern Med 1986;146:2365-7.

Blower AL. Considerations for nonsteroidal anti-inflammatory drug therapy safety Scandinavian Journal of Rheumatology 1996;25:13-26.

Coles LS, Fries JF, Draines RG, et al. From experiment to experience: Side effects of NSAIDs. Am J Med 1983;74:820-8.

Dajani EZ, Agrawal NM. NSAID-induced gastrointestinal damage in the elderly. Intern Med Specialist 1990;11:91-110.

Delmas PD. Non-steroidal anti-inflammatory drugs and renal function. British Journal of Rheumatology 1995;34:25-28.

Fries J. Toward an understanding of NSAID-related adverse events: The contribution of longitudinal data. Scandinavian Journal of Rheumatology 1996;25:3-8.

Fries JF, Miller SR, Spitz PW, et al. Toward an epidemiology of gastropathy associated with nonsteroidal anti-inflammatory drug use. Gastroenterology 1989;96:647-55.

Hawkey CJ. Non-steroidal anti-inflammatory drug gastropathy: causes and treatment. Scandinavian Journal of Gastroenterology 1996;220:124-7.

Emery P. Clinical implications of selective cyclooxygenase-2 inhibition. Scandinavian Journal of Rheumatology 1996;25:23-28.

Simon LS, Hatoum HT, Bittman RM, et al. Risk factors for serious nonsteroidal-induced gastrointestinal complications: regression analysis of the MUCOSA trial. Family Medicine 1996; 28:204-10.

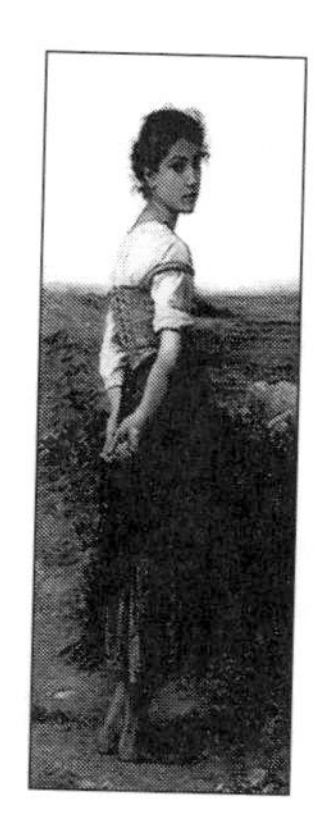

Chapter 5
Four Patients With Shoulder Pain

"I have been friends with Marc (Darrow) forever, and because many of our acquaintances had been healed by Prolotherapy, I thought I would give it a shot (no pun intended.)

After the first set of injections, for a day or so, my shoulder felt like someone had punched it. I was reluctant to be injected again. Then on a trip with Marc and some friends, while he was injecting them, he said I needed to be injected one more time. I agreed, and to my surprise, my shoulder was healed completely within the next couple of days."

Jsu Garcia

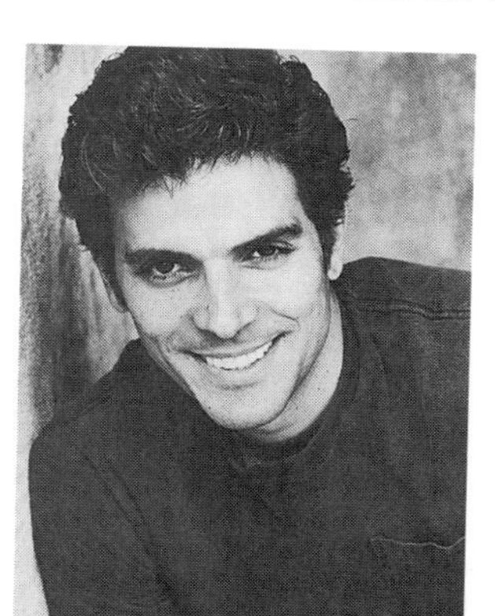

Jsu Garcia

When you are an actor and have to stand in the same camera frame with Arnold Schwarzenegger or Mel Gibson, you would want to look your best physically—to be able to "hold your own" on-screen with these Hollywood hunks.

This is exactly what Jsu Garcia thought. So when his agent told him he would be appearing opposite Arnold in "Collateral Damage," Jsu began training.

"I did vigorous 'boot camp' activity for weeks and 680 push-ups a day," says Jsu. "My shoulder finally gave out, (and) it just wouldn't heal. I hurt myself really bad."

What happened to Jsu, happens to many.

The Leading Causes of Shoulder Pain

Repetitive overhead sports motions, such as pitching, swimming, or the tennis serve;

-Heavy lifting;
-Excessive force, such as a fall;
-Degeneration due to aging;
-Narrowing of the space (acromioclavicular joint) between the collarbone (clavicle) and the top portion (acromion) of the shoulder bone (scapula);
-Abrasion of the rotator cuff surface by the top portion of the shoulder bone (the acromium).

Injury To The Shoulder

The shoulder is really a combination of several joints—combined in such a way by an intricate arrangement of muscles and tendons—that provides the arm a wide range of motion, flexibility and stability.

The rotator cuff is a group of four shoulder muscles that surround the top of the upper arm bone, the humerus, and holds it

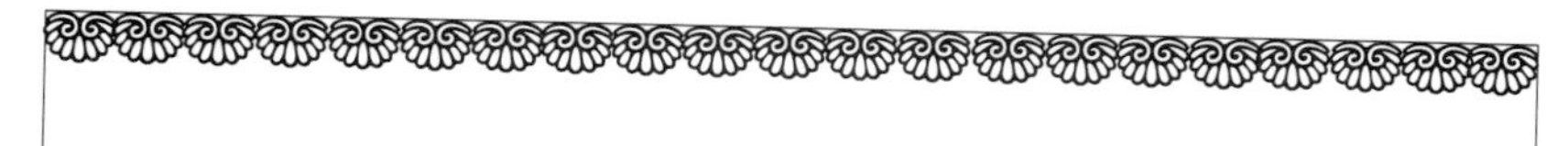

in the shoulder joint. These muscles are responsible for moving the arm in various directions, and unlike the massive deltoid muscle of the upper arm, are smaller and generally more vulnerable to injury. The four muscles and tendons of the rotator cuff are the supraspinatus, infraspinatus, teres minor, and sub scapularis. It is the supraspinatus that is most commonly inflamed or torn.

The supraspinatus, and the rest of the shoulder, because they are built and expected to allow a remarkable array of motion, frequently are subjected to the injuries listed above, causing problems of instability or impingement of soft tissue and pain. The pain may be constant, or may occur only when the shoulder is moved. In any case, any shoulder pain that persists more than a few days should be diagnosed and treated as necessary.

Shoulder Inflammation/Tendinitis

Tendinitis in the shoulder is often an inflammation of the tendons as a result of the wearing process that takes place over a period of time. It can also occur from an unusual, awkward movement or fall.

Sometimes, excessive use or injury of the shoulder leads to inflammation and swelling of a bursa, a condition known as bursitis.

Bursas are fluid filled sacs located around the body and joints. They lessen the friction caused by movement of the shoulder. Bursitis often occurs in association with rotator cuff tendinitis. Symptoms of shoulder bursitis include mild to severe pain, limiting the use of the shoulder. In extreme cases the joint stiffens into a condition known as "frozen shoulder," also referred to by doctors as adhesive capsulitis.

Shoulder Impingement Syndrome

Shoulder impingement syndrome involves one or a combination of problems: inflammation of the bursa located just over the rotator cuff, inflammation of the rotator cuff tendons (tendinitis), or calcium deposits in tendons—called calcific tendonitis, (caused by wear and tear or injury.) The main problem is usually that the acromium or a bone spur puts pressure on the supraspinatus tendon.

Chronic Shoulder Instability Syndrome

Chronic shoulder instability syndrome results from trauma caused by subluxations, dislocations, from less detectable micro-trauma caused by repetitive strain, or from congenitally loose shoulder joints. Recurrent pain or tenderness in the shoulder joint and weakness in the arm are two of the more common symptoms, but severe examples include patients whose shoulders pop in and out of joint. Frequent shoulder dislocations stretch the brachial plexus, the nerves that run from the neck down the arm. This process can cause permanent nerve damage, pain, and loss of use of the arm.

Shoulder Dislocations

Sometimes the bones in the shoulder joint slip out of normal alignment or are forced out by injury, a condition known as subluxation—if partial in nature, and dislocation—if completely out of joint.

Most shoulder sprains or, more seriously, dislocations happen when a person falls on an outstretched hand, or sustains a blow to the shoulder (especially a downward blow.)

Approximately 95% of shoulder dislocations are anterior dislocations, in which the anterior static shoulder stabilizers are stretched or torn away from the bone.

Until recently it was common in cases of dislocation to immobilize the shoulder for long periods of time. But studies proved that while immobilization helped alleviate the pain of such injuries, it also contributed to a general weakening of the ligaments and predominance of adhesive capsulitis.

In one alarming study of close to 250 patients, about half of those treated with immobilization had recurring dislocations

within the 10 year period of the study. The problem is greater in younger people. This is one of the few areas where older folks have an advantage, because their connective tissues are less elastic, the risk of dislocation is less likely.

Shoulder Arthritis

There are many types of arthritis, but most often in the shoulder it is triggered by an initial trauma.

It can also involve "wear and tear" of the tissues of the joint, causing inflammation, swelling and pain.

Often people will react by instinctively limiting their shoulder movements in order to lessen the pain. This can lead to a tightening or stiffening of the soft tissue parts of the joint, resulting in yet further pain and restriction of motion. In the worst cases, adhesive capsulitis occurs and the arm can not be moved.

Referred Pain

The musculature of the shoulder area is fertile ground for trigger points, as is evidenced by the prevalence of a "stiff neck" and referred pain radiating anteriorly, laterally or posteriorly from all three of the major scalene muscles into the arms, chest or vertebrae. Trigger points from the trapezius muscles can refer pain to the head and down the arms.

Okay, You Know About the Problems and Pain, Now What?

If you are one of the more than four million people in the United States who seek medical care each year for shoulder problems, a brief understanding of the treatment options may help you decide what many already know. Prolotherapy may be your permanent answer, as Jsu Garcia found out.

"I couldn't do any kind of chest lifting, (because) it was sore. It was a three month thing...kicking me really hard, and now it's gone, I'm back, I can lift weights."

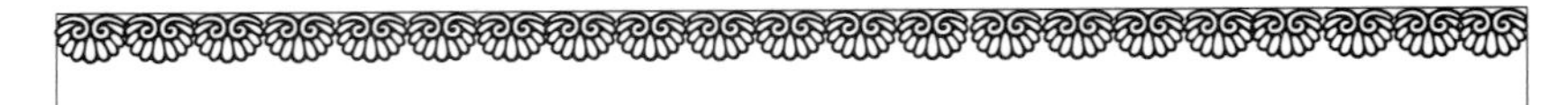

A proper diagnosis of shoulder pain is essential to determine the root cause of the problem and the proper method of treatment. Because many shoulder conditions are caused by specific activities, such as Jsu Garcia's over-use caused by excessive workouts, a detailed medical history is an invaluable tool.

A physical examination should also include screening for physical abnormalities—swelling, deformity, muscle weakness, and tender areas—and observing the range of shoulder motion—how far and in which directions the arm can be moved.

Although x-rays may be helpful in defining problems, more elusive ones may require computerized tomography (CT scan), which provides a more detailed view of the bones. Electrodiagnostic studies such as the electromyogram (EMG) and a nerve conduction study can indicate whether pain or weakness in the area is coming from a pinched nerve in the neck, or a peripheral nerve injury away from the neck, or down the arm. Magnetic Resonance Imaging (MRI) and ultrasound are other safe and effective diagnostic tools, providing images of the soft tissues without using radiation. An arthrogram is an x-ray, CT or MRI in which dye is injected into the joint for added contrast. However, as outlined in other sections of this book, studies have shown that the advanced technologies commonly used to diagnosis injuries are grievously insufficient to show where the pain is coming from.

This is when a Prolotherapist and his ability to reproduce pain by touching is invaluable. If you can put your finger on the exact spot that is causing the pain, then there is a high probability that you are a candidate for shoulder Prolotherapy since most shoulder problems involve the soft tissues—muscles, ligaments, and tendons—rather than the bones. As outlined earlier in this

Since it's been proven to strengthen the connective tissues, and has the benefit of over fifty years of testing, Prolotherapy is arguably one of the best choices of treatment in cases of dislocation, rotator cuff tendonitis, bursitis, muscle tissue impingement or recurring instability.

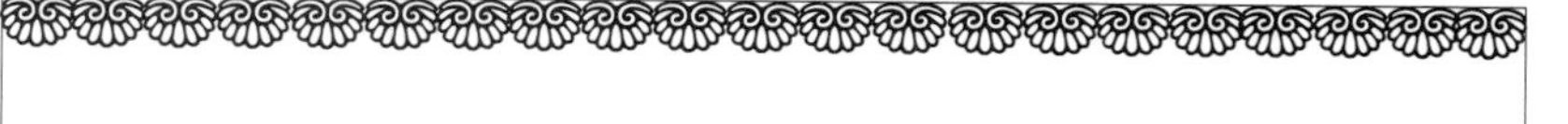

book, these soft tissue injuries are precisely the kinds of injury that respond so effectively to Prolotherapy.

Many of the structures inside of joints that are injured do not hurt when you press on the outer surfaces. These inner structures can often be healed with Prolotherapy.

Before you do anything as radical or irreversible as surgery, and before you accept the grim prognosis of conventional medicine that sentences you to a lifetime of dependence on pain relief medication, you owe it to yourself to try Prolotherapy, as another Hollywood star, Jessica Tuck did.

Jessica was in excruciating pain while on the set of the CBS show, "Judging Amy," then, as she says, "the magic happened." Here is her story...

Jessica Tuck, Star of Judging Amy

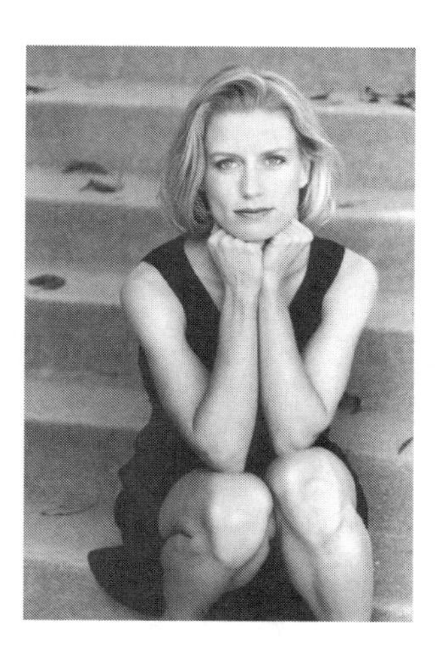

Jessica Tuck

"I came to Joint Rehab because of a referral from a friend. She told me that Prolotherapy injections could help my shoulder pain.

My left shoulder bothered me on and off for more than a year. The last two months prior to coming to Dr. Darrow was a period of escalating, excruciating pain. On the show (*Judging Amy*), I was carrying a 21-month-old baby for extended periods of time.

I normally do yoga, hiking, and I roller-blade, but sports came to a standstill because of pain.

I found out that I was doing yoga 'wrong' which also exacerbated the pain. Dr. Darrow's staff showed me how to do it the right way.

After the first two Prolotherapy sessions, my shoulder ached for a day, and I was a little concerned that it wasn't working.

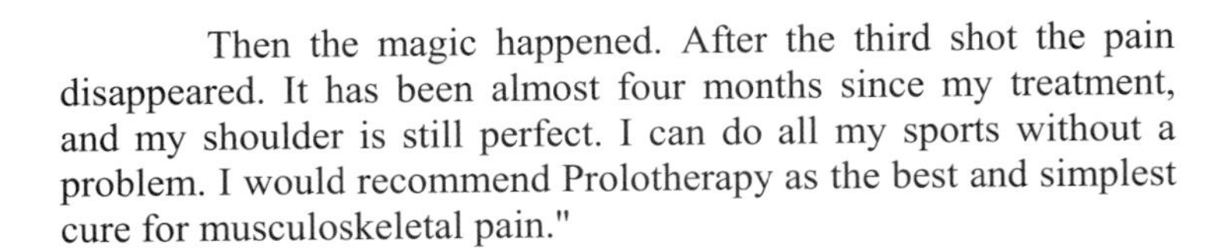

Then the magic happened. After the third shot the pain disappeared. It has been almost four months since my treatment, and my shoulder is still perfect. I can do all my sports without a problem. I would recommend Prolotherapy as the best and simplest cure for musculoskeletal pain."

Frank Cassavetes

Frank Cassavetes is not only an actor and personal trainer to some of Hollywood's superstars, he is also a hero. A marine veteran of 27 years, with 29 months in combat in Viet Nam. Captured, he was a prisoner of war for five years, the last three at the infamous Hanoi Hilton prisoner of war camp.

Due to the physical cruelty he experienced as a POW, many of his joints were permanently injured, leaving him in severe, chronic pain.

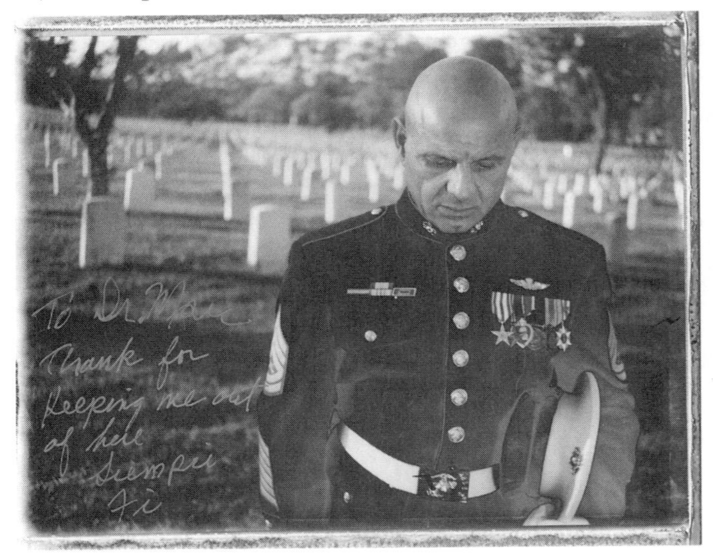

Frank Cassavetes

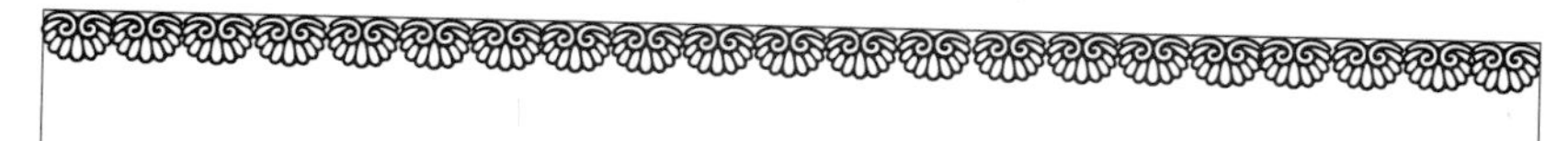

For the last ten years of his military career, Frank was a drill instructor at the Marine training camp at Parris Island.

Most will recognize Frank as the sniper in the movie "John Q" with Denzel Washington, who Frank also worked with as a personal trainer.

At the time of this writing, Frank was getting ready for roles in movies with Michael Caine, Robert Duval, and his brother, the well-known producer Nick Cassavetes.

"Beside acting, I am a personal trainer at Gold's Gym. I train lots of different people, professional fighters, professional athletes, actors," says Frank.

"And for years I have had a lot of problems with my joints. The worst was my whole shoulder area. My spinatus, supraspinatus, and levator scapular area, the whole area, I couldn't even hold my arm up.

Marc (Dr. Darrow) convinced me that Prolotherapy could help. I started coming into the office once a week for six weeks for the shots. Suddenly, it was like, I'm a new man. I was able to train and box again."

Jonathan Haze, Cult Movie Legend

Classic Roger Corman horror movie fans need no introduction to Jonathan Haze, the star of such cult classics as "Little Shop of Horrors." The actor, now in his mid-70's, can now be seen frequently on television commercials.

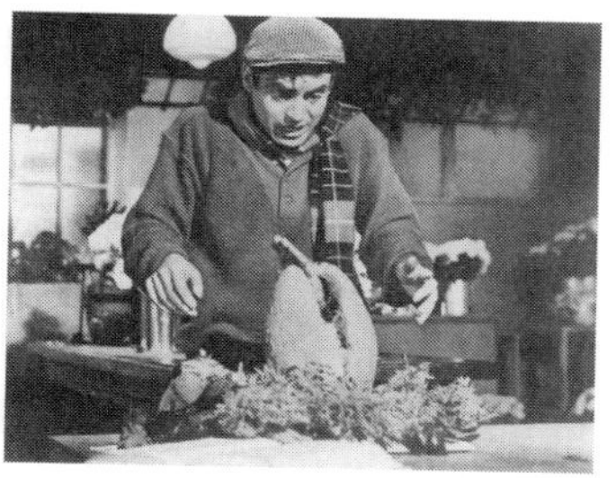

A car accident caused Jonathan numerous pains, most intensely in his shoulder. Jonathan is no ordinary 70-ish year-old. As an actor, he keeps himself busy with commercial work, and to maintain his appearance, a strict body-building schedule. Shoulder pain has no place in his life.

"In January 2001, I was driving my little Porsche over Laurel Canyon to go to an audition. Some guy in a pick-up truck going in the other direction lost control and spun out and smashed into the driver's side of my car, right into the door which my shoulder was right up against. The impact of the crash then threw me the other way, which snapped my neck and back. So, I went to a lawyer and they sent me to see an orthopedic surgeon who sent me to have physical therapy for about two weeks, which was pleasant, but I don't think that it really helped. I still had the pain."

Jonathan relays that he had other less successful treatments as well.

"I had two cortisone shots. The first cortisone shot was like a miracle. It was 'instant no pain' and lasted for about two months. Then, when the pain came back, I went and had another one and it was the same thing. I saw Dr. Murray Susser who suggested I see Dr. Darrow for Prolotherapy."

As with many new patients to Prolotherapy, Jonathan tells a story similar to those above of Jsu's and Jessica's first encounter with Prolotherapy.

"The first shot was pretty scary, because it's a long needle and I got six or eight injections, but, I had an anesthetic and didn't feel any real pain. However, two days later it was sore!"

Also like many new Prolotherapy patients, Jonathan quickly began to see results.

"About two days after that, suddenly the pain started to ease off and I felt great. Still a little pain, but much better. Much better movement, and much less pain. So after the first treatment it was much better. Now after five treatments I am claiming about 90-95% improvement because that's how good it feels!"

Jonathan's Prolotherapy treatment also helped him avoid the surgeon's knife. "I had two doctors tell me that I should have surgery. The first doctor told me that the pain in my shoulder was coming from my neck and he was going to operate on that. The second doctor said that he could clean up my rotator cuff really nice with arthroscopic surgery. As soon as I hear surgery I leave.

I would definitely recommend it for anybody with any kind of pain, as the first thing to go to. There is no reason for any surgery, there really isn't. I have already recommended Prolotherapy to various people."

References

Travell JG, Simmons DG. Myofascial Pain and Dysfunction: The Trigger Point Manual. Williams and Wilkins;1983:334.

Mayo Clinic Women's Health Source, December 8, 2000.

Wheaton M (contributor). Prolo Your Sports Injuries Away!, Hauser R, Hauser M. Beulah Land Press; Oak Park, 2001:252.

Havelius L. Anterior Dislocations of the Shoulder in Teenagers and Young Adults. American Journal of Bone and Joint Surgery;1987;69:393-399.

Advances in Sports Medicine, American Academy of Orthopaedic Surgeons (AAOS), October 18, 2000.

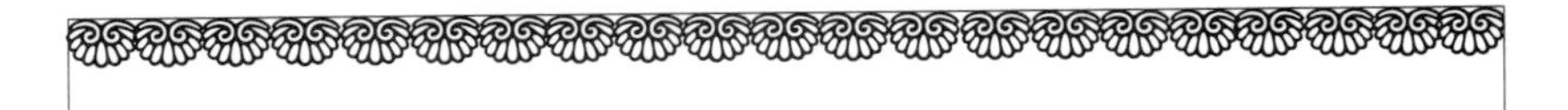

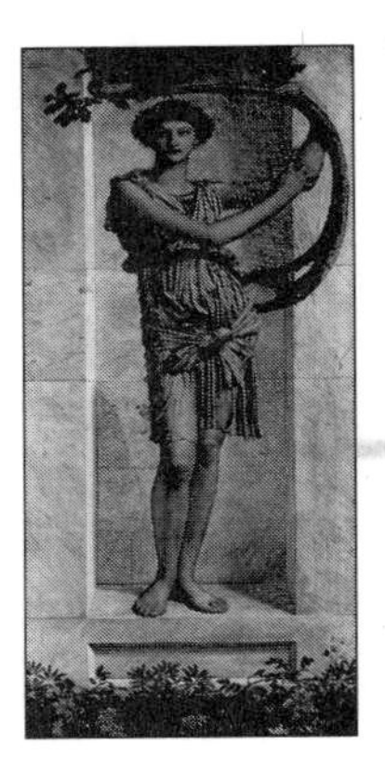

"To wish to be well is part of becoming well"
—Seneca—

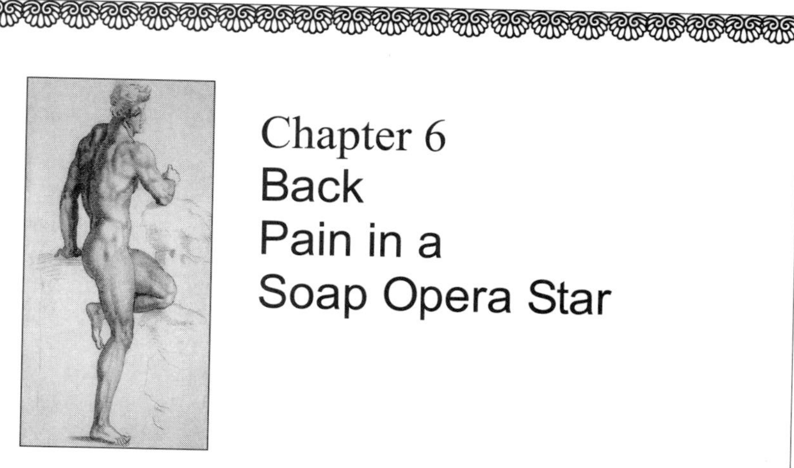

Chapter 6 Back Pain in a Soap Opera Star

"I was told that I needed immediate surgery. To help with the pain I was given repeated epidural injections with steroids and told I would probably never be off Vicodin (a narcotic pain killer.) Specialist after specialist told me that I should not even be walking around, my discs could rupture at any time!"

It could have been a scene from many of the scripts Emmy-nominated actress Amy Gibson has read in her years on the "Young & The Restless", "General Hospital", and "Love of Life."

A young beautiful woman is told by seven doctors that she has several herniated and two bulging discs and needs an operation immediately to prevent her from being confined to a wheel chair.

The catch, they told her, is that the surgery is so risky that it in itself carries a 50-50% chance of causing enough damage to confine her to a wheelchair for life.

Unfortunately for Amy this was not a script, this was the reality of a succession of sports injuries, car accidents and poor chiropractic care.

Back Pain

Eighty percent of Americans suffer from back pain at some point.

One out of 10 people in the United States is actively seeking health care for back pain. It is the most common cause of industrial disability and the leading cause of physical disability payments taxing our Social Security system.

Most Lower Back Pain is From a Sprain of the Sacroiliac and Iliolumbar Ligaments

In medical terminology, "acute" pain means new pain, it does not refer to severity.

"Chronic" is the term usually reserved for pain lasting longer than three months, often involving psychological (such as stress) as well as physical factors, or combinations of the two.

As with all types of pain, there are many possible factors causing or contributing to both the acute and chronic types of lower back pain.

However, damage to the ligaments of the back is estimated to be responsible for up to 70% of all cases of lower back pain. In my clinic, I would estimate these causes to be as high as 95% of back pain.

The chronic back pain patient typically experiences some type of trauma to the lower back that causes injury to the iliolumbar, sacroiliac, interspinous and supraspinous ligaments.

Over a long period of time this may cause some forward slippage of the fifth lumbar vertebra from the sacrum, which in turn causes excessive pressure on the vertebral disc. Fissures may occur in the disc (at the annulus fibrosis), and this exacerbates the degenerative disc problem.

Amy's story of back pain started in 1993 when she injured her knee and tail bone in a water skiing accident. This incident was followed by a series of car accidents that further aggravated her condition. "I also played a lot of golf and tennis, something I guess

**REFERRED PAIN AND SCIATICA–
ILIOLUMBAR, POSTERIOR SACROILIAC, SACROSPINUS AND SACROTUBERUS LIGAMENTS .
(LUMBOSACRAL AND SACROILIAC JOINT INSTABILITY.)**

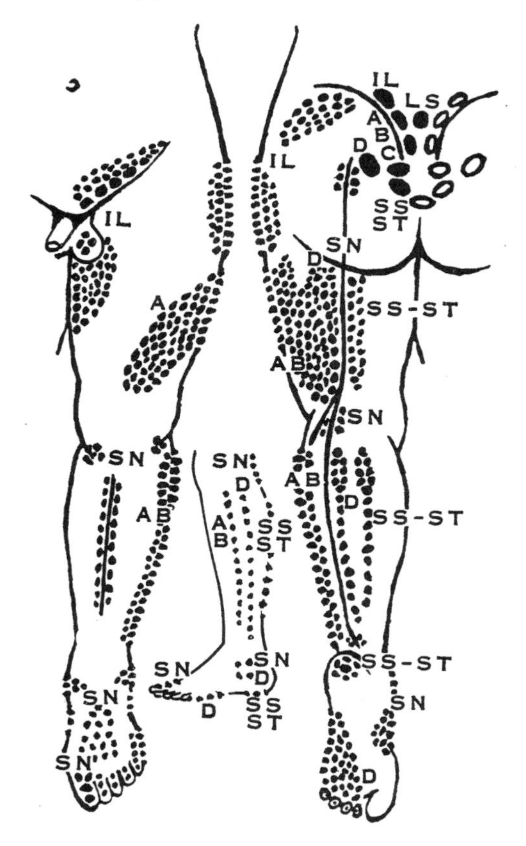

FIGURE 9. REFERRED PAIN OF ILIOLUMBAR, POSTERIOR SACROILIAC, SACROSPINUS AND SACROTUBERUS LIGAMENTS, AND SCIATICA.
Referred pain areas from the iliolumbar (Fig. 2-IL) and sacroiliac (Fig. 3-A,B,C,D), articular supporting ligaments (Fig. 4-SS-ST), along with the conducted pain of sciatica (Fig. 5-SN) are combined in one dermatome.

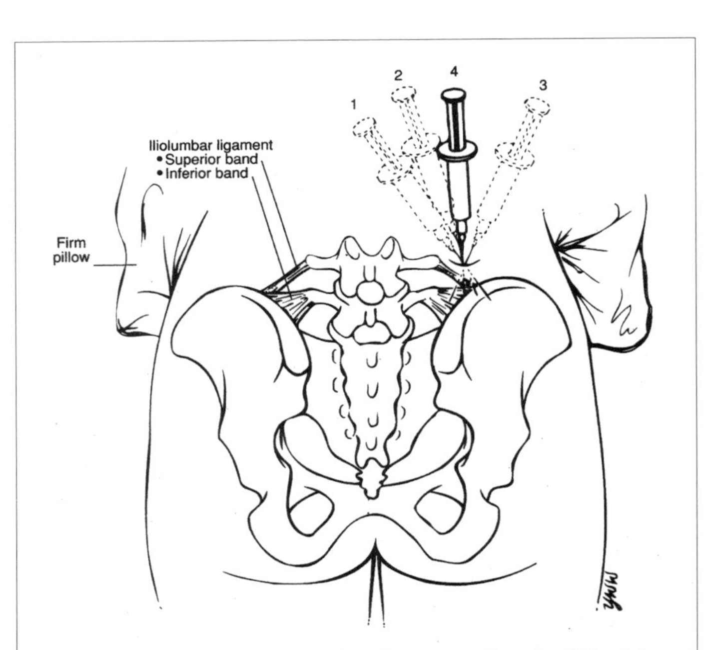

Fig. 3.9 Injection of the iliolumbar ligament using the "Hirschberg technique." The needle contacts the superior aspect of the iliac crest and is then advanced over the anterior margins. When the needle drops over the anterior aspect of the iliac crest, the physician is certain of the needle position, and the needle is then redirected back onto the superior aspect of the crest for injection of 5 cc of the dextrose proliferant solution. A firm pillow under the patient's abdomen makes palpation and injection easier.

some one with a bad back shouldn't do." After poor chiropractic treatment Amy was basically bedridden for over a year.

Ligament Laxity

Ligaments are designed to handle a normal amount of stress (activity or injury) that will stretch them to their natural limit. Once the stress is removed, the ligaments return to their normal length. If additional (traumatic) stress is applied—stretching the

ligament beyond its natural range of extension—the ligament will not return to its normal length, but will instead remain permanently over-stretched, diminishing its ability to hold the vertebrae in their proper place. Such a condition is called "ligament laxity."

Ligament laxity in the lower back, as elsewhere in the body, maybe caused by a major traumatic injury, repeated minor injuries to the same area, simple normal aging, or wearing out the collagen. As explained earlier in this book, because of poor blood supply, ligaments do not heal well on their own, so once laxity exists, pain is only one wrong turn, twist or exertion away. Prolotherapy stimulates the rejuvenation and tightening of these lax ligaments. Many people with this problem have intermittent periods of low back pain that increases with frequency and in severity with aging.

Back Surgery

"Because of the imminent threat of rupture, the doctors kept pushing me towards surgery. But the chance of poor surgical outcome was so high, I sought an alternative treatment. I decided on Prolotherapy," said Amy.

Failed back syndrome is an official-sounding term to describe the pain of patients whose surgical attempts have failed to correct their back pain problems.

The most common cause of failed back syndrome is poor judgment on the part of the physician. This poor judgment is based on surgery prescribed as a last resort—on a hope and a prayer—that it might alleviate the pain.

Often surgery is done because of the wrong diagnosis. Unfortunately, often times surgery does little to help, and, in fact, can make things worse. Frequently surgery results in post-operative scarring, which often exacerbates the initial problem or causes new pain syndromes.

The MRI can show a herniated disc that has been present and asymptomatic for years.

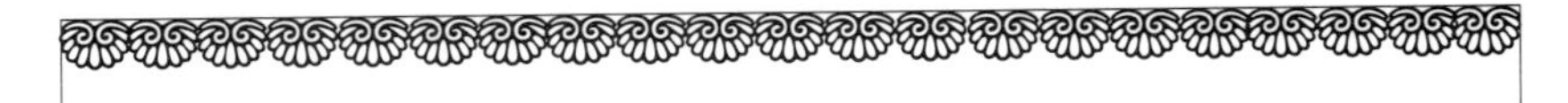

The surgeon fixes the asymptomatic disc but the pain of the lax ligaments persist.

Subsequent "corrective" surgery can help in some cases, particularly if the damage done by the first operation involves clearly observable physical complications like nerve root compression, massive scarring, bone spurring or foraminal compression.

Unfortunately, the rate of success for second surgical operations in the case of "failed back syndrome" is no greater than it was for the initial operation, and declines with further attempts.

Prolotherapy to the Rescue

Can Prolotherapy really fix a back problem where surgery can not? Many are skeptical including Amy Gibson, once.

"I was sold on Prolotherapy but still remained skeptical. Especially since I was being told that a simple injection treatment could safely do what a major spinal surgery probably couldn't. But after the fourth treatment, (normally a patient receives three to six treatment sessions), I noticed an incredible improvement."

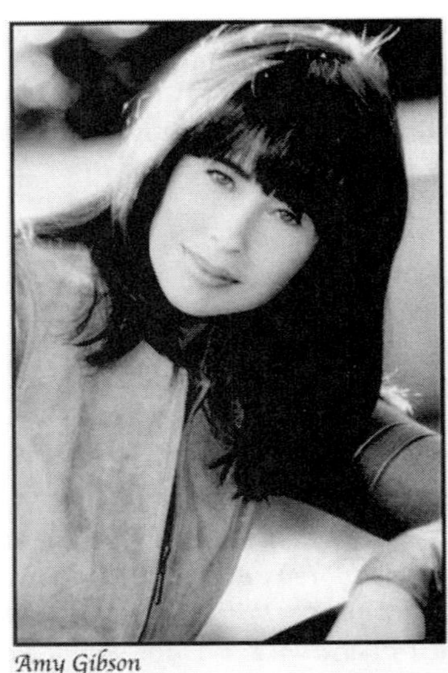

Amy Gibson

A study published in 1987[1]—by which time the procedures of Prolotherapy were fairly well established—offered dramatic support to proponents of the still basically unknown technique. In the first double-blind study on the effects of Prolotherapy on back pain, two groups of carefully screened patients—with at least a one

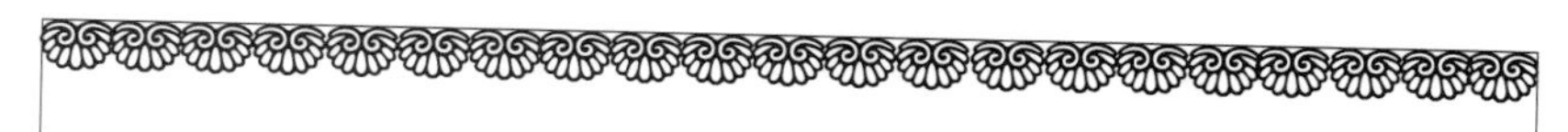

year history of back problems that had not responded to other non-surgical treatments—were injected with either a true Prolotherapy proliferant (a dextrose-glycerine-phenol solution), or with a saline-based placebo.

The test subjects had been thoroughly pre-screened, with full clinical evaluations, x-rays and lab tests, and the 82 patients accepted had arrived with painful conditions. Sixty-percent were currently using non-steroidal anti-inflammatory drugs (NSAIDs). A half-dozen were experiencing such intense pain that they were taking narcotic painkillers. A whopping 91% had difficulty sitting still for any length of time, and 65% had difficulty sleeping due to their pain. Seventeen-percent had difficulty walking, 21% experienced decreased sexual activity, and 4% were completely bed-ridden.

Six months after the treatment, 35 of the 40 people who had received the actual Prolotherapy treatment had experienced at least a 50% reduction in pain—a success rate of 88%. And 15 of them were completely pain free compared to only 4 in the control group.

Other "pain score" indicators backed up the results of this data, confirming the success of the therapy. One thing was eminently clear: Prolotherapy worked for the treatment of chronic low back pain.

Amy Gibson did not need a scientific study to validate the effectiveness of Prolotherapy to her.

"I had an audition in New York. It is a day I will always remember. I was staying at 57th Street and 8th Avenue and decided to walk to 23rd Street for my audition (about two miles.) I told myself that if I could walk to this audition, I was really able to work again, and I made it!

"I walked into this audition and the director asked me why I was so sweaty. I told him that I had walked there from 57th

Ligament and Tendon Relaxation

TRIGGER POINTS OF PAIN AND NEEDLES IN POSITION FOR CONFIRMATION OF THE DIAGNOSIS AND FOR TREATMENT OF LIGAMENT RELAXATION OF THE LUMBOSACRAL AND PELVIC JOINTS.
TRIGGER POINTS OF LIGAMENTS

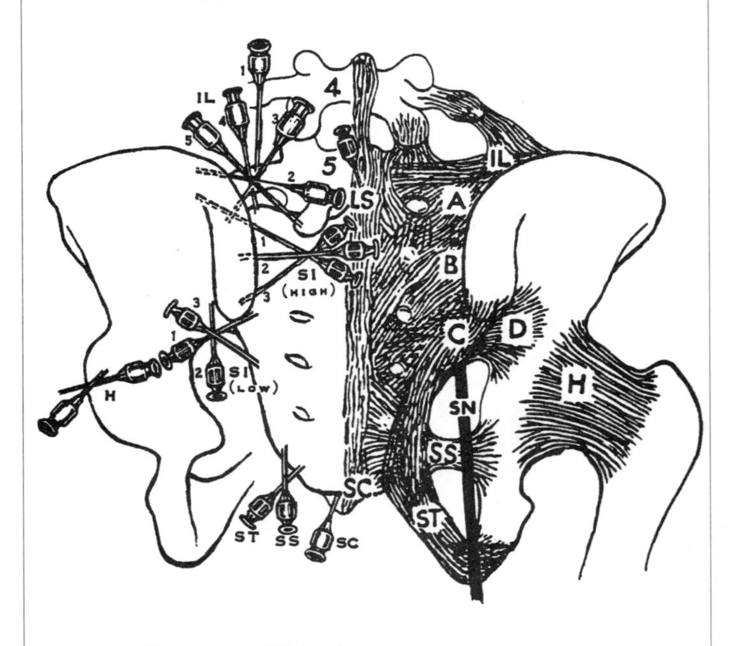

IL	-	**Iliolumbar**
LS	-	**Lumbosacral - Supra & Interspinus**
A,B,C,D,-		**Posterior Sacroiliac**
SS	-	**Sacrospinus**
ST	-	**Sacrotuberus**
SC	-	**Sacrococcygeal**
H	-	**Hip - Articular**
SN	-	**Sciatic nerve**

FIGURE 1.

Street. To a New Yorker that is no big deal so he said, 'Oh, that's nice.' I said, 'No, you don't understand, I WALKED here.' He asked, 'So am I missing something?' Then I told him the story and he said, 'Wow, that is so cool that you walked here. By the way, I got the part!'"

The Role of Chiropractic and Prolotherapy

Amy Gibson's back problems were exacerbated by poor chiropractic care. Poor chiropractic care is certainly not the norm. In our clinic, we are pleased to have one of the best chiropractors available for our patients, Jason Kelberman, D.C.

Dr. Kelberman sometimes utilizes a chiropractic method called Applied Kinesiology (AK), in cases of back pain, injury, or post-surgery because it does not involve "cracking" the vertebrae.

I am fond of saying chiropractic is the same as Prolotherapy without the needles.

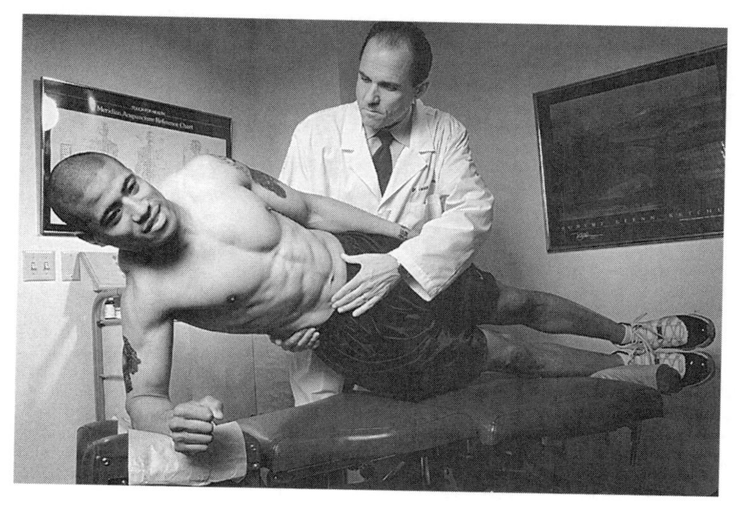

Dr. Kelberman applies chiropractic treatment to NFL wide receiver Johnnie Morton

Both treatments desire to do the same thing, put the vertebrae or any joint back in the place it belongs. The difference however is that chiropractic adjustment may only provide temporary relief because it cannot correct the underlying cause of back pain, ligament laxity. This is what Prolotherapy does. The triad of Prolotherapy, chiropractic, and MedX (to be discussed next) is the key to our success.

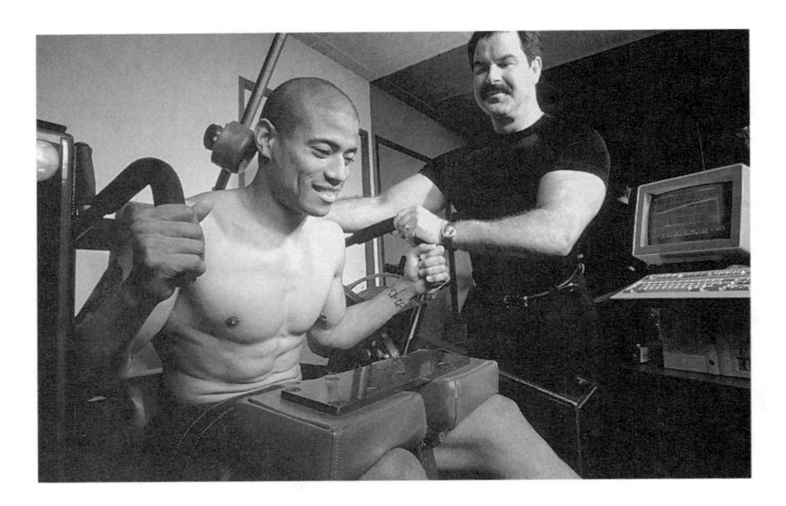

Johnnie Morton getting the MedX Back Strengthening workout from

Exercises for the Back

Another highly successful therapy that ***Joint Rehabilitation & Sports Medical Center, Inc.*** employs is MedX. Frequently, back and neck injuries occur from structural weakness. Studies by prominent orthopedic surgeons have proven that MedX strengthens the back and neck, alleviates pain, and prevents surgery.

MedX is a computerized back & neck strengthening machine that tests the exact level of weakness and then provides a built in therapy that brings those areas to optimal strength.

A MedX workout twice a week for several weeks has been proven to be so effective that it is covered by insurance and Medicare.

A person using the machine sits upright in a chair while several pads and belts exert pressure on the thighs and hips to prevent them from moving. Then a weight is determined through a static testing procedure and an exercise protocol is designed for each patient's needs. The goal is to increase strength levels and active range of motion to get the patient back to full function in their daily activities. MedX is designed to isolate the paraspinal muscles that stabilize the spine.

Why then surgically fix the spine with bone or metal when it can be done with exercise, Prolotherapy, and chiropractic?

In 1999, a two year follow-up study of 60 patients with a surgical diagnosis, showed that only two went on to have surgery after MedX Rehabilitation.

Our clinic is lucky to have one of the top MedX exercise physiologists in the world, Dr. Bill Bergman, PhD. Dr. Bergman studied under the MedX inventor, Arthur Jones, who also invented Nautilus® exercise equipment.

Over the past 12 years, he has trained well over 10,000 patients. In this group he has seen professional bodybuilders, football players, wrestlers, surfers, volleyball players, golfers, Olympic athletes, track and field participants, martial artists, and the list goes on. They are among the best athletes in the world but still tested below what is considered a healthy back and neck strength for their ages, weight and gender. These areas just aren't addressed in training programs. With this in mind, just consider how important MedX is for the less active person.

A case history involving tennis pro Jim Pugh illustrates the benefits that MedX can provide. Pugh, an eight-time grand slam winner, came to our clinic and saw Jason Kelberman, D.C.

Pugh was suffering from low back pain which had plagued him for three months, leaving him unable to play or teach tennis.

Dr. Kelberman determined that his restricted range of motion and diminished strength were consistent with degenerative disc syndrome. After only three sessions of chiropractic adjustments, Dr. Kelberman was able to significantly reduce Pugh's pain, at which point he had Pugh begin a strengthening program using the MedX. The result was that Pugh's strength quickly improved and he was able to again play tennis at competitive levels.

With a combination of Prolotherapy, chiropractic care, MedX, and an intensive rehabilitation program that focuses on stretching, elimination of local inflammatory changes, spinal muscle strengthening, and general reconditioning, most patients improve by increasing function and mobility, and decreasing pain.

The Role of Psychological Factors in Back Pain

There is much to be said for reducing the stress load in one's life when trying to deal with chronic back pain. (Refer back to Chapter 4).

Stanford University researchers studied 96 people with high-risk factors for disc degeneration, to measure the psychological factors on back pain. Surprisingly they found that people at high-risk for disc degeneration were only slightly more likely to experience back pain during normal activity than people without obvious disc problems. In fact, 25 percent of the high-risk group had no corresponding symptoms of low back pain!

This meant to the Stanford researchers that doctors should know that damaged discs do not automatically mean that the patient is experiencing pain, and also if pain is present, surgery will not necessarily eliminate it because of the stress factors in the patient's life.

A better predictor of pain, they found, is an abnormal result on psychometric testing. Basically, that the amount of discomfort that people have is related to their ability to handle stress. Says

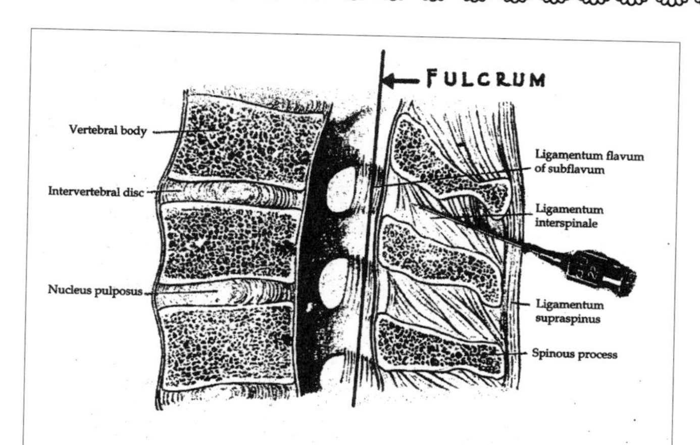

Fig. 13. Vertical section through lumbar vertebrae. Vertical line passes through the two articular fulcrums. One and one-half inch needle in position for confirmation of the diagnosis and for treatment.

The point of the needle has passed through the supraspinus ligament and is in the *diagonal* fibers of the interspinus ligament.

When one vertebra normally glides forward on the articular processes of the adjoining vertebra below, both the interspinus and supraspinus ligaments assume a more diagonal position without stretching, as the spines of the two vertebrae come slightly closer together.

To permit any abnormal forward movement of one vertebra on another such as occurs in spondylolisthesis and compressing an intervertebral disc, the fibers of the interspinus ligament must be torn or stretched, as in chronic relaxation, while the supraspinus ligament may assume a more diagonal position in the moderate cases but must also be disabled together with the spinus articular ligaments and others in the severe cases.

The interspinus ligaments are probably the most important ligament throughout the spine in limiting joint motion while maintaining joint stability.

The interspinus relaxation is frequently accompanied by relaxation of the articular ligaments on one or both sides of the same vertebra.

lead Stanford researcher Dr. Eugene Carragee, "People with poor coping skills...are more likely to perceive discography as painful and to have symptoms of low back pain during their daily activities."

The results suggest that physicians must be acutely aware of the emotional or psychological factors that may be affecting how patients perceive their back pain.

Carragee believes it is vital to the patient's recovery to get to the true root of the problem, which may have both physical and

emotional dimensions. It is especially important to avoid unnecessary, invasive and expensive treatments, such as back fusions, that reinforce the perception that the patient has a grave disease of the spine.

As many as 30,000 back fusions are performed annually in the United States, Carragee estimates, although they are often not very successful at relieving the patient's pain. Believe it or not, more than 400,000 back surgeries are performed each year in the United States.

Other Back Problems Helped By Prolotherapy

- **Lumbosacral strain or sprain** indicates a soft tissue injury of the lower back, equivalent in a sense to a sprained ankle.

- **Discogenic Syndrome** is used to describe pain originating in the lumbar disc, often due to tears in the annulus, release of chemical mediators, or micromotion.

- **Disc Herniation** indicates a displacement of the nucleus pulposus from the intervertebral space into the spinal canal or foramen, or outside the foramen. This can "pinch" a nerve root and cause sciatica.

- **Facet Syndrome** describes pain originating in the zygapophyseal or "facet" joints between the vertebrae, characteristically localized in the back, aggravated by movement and alleviated by rest.

- **Spondylolisthesis** is the slipping forward, or backward, of one vertebral segment over another. Retrolisthesis describes the slipping backward of one vertebra over another. Anterolisthesis describes the slipping forward of a vertebra over another.

- **Spondylolysis** indicates a defect in the structure of the pars interarticularis.

- **Spondylosis** is a catch-all phrase describing the arthritic changes that occur as a result of degenerative disc disease, narrowing of the interspace, inflammation, spurring or degeneration of the bone, and ligament hypertrophy.
- **Degenerative Disc Disease** refers to the desiccation (drying out) of the vertebral discs. When this occurs, the discs often shrink or collapse and the vertebrae move closer together. This can cause ligament laxity.

- **Spinal Stenosis** is used to describe the narrowing, in part or in whole, of the spinal canal, either through spondylolsis or a congenital defect.

- **Spinal Instability** refers to excess motion of the vertebrae and can be shown on flexion and extension x-rays. If instability is severe, it can cause spinal cord injury and paralysis. In more benign cases, it simply causes pain.

A Unique Case-Fusion Surgery Avoided Martin Hyman's Story

"I'm 72 now and feel great. Yet, in my lifetime I have been offered five surgeries, radiation, and lots of pills, often with weird side effects.

Over a period of 50 years I've dealt successfully with severe low back problems, ulcers, prostate cancer, and an ominous family history of heart disease.

In each case I looked for another idea and resisted getting stampeded into predictable treatment. I read a lot and interviewed doctors. I would even call the author of a book or article on the subject. I always ask the same question. What is the minority opinion of a treatment and who are they? Who are these doctors that are literally going against the flow? Each time I found the maverick, the individualist with the courage to go his own way. Often they were insulted by colleagues, refused publication, and denied an audience.

The success I experienced in going against the common way of thinking in other battles set me up for resolving what had been a dominating problem since the age of 19 when I hurt my low back in a factory lifting accident.

Two top orthopedic surgeons recommended fusion surgery and my folks and I declined. The next 20 years was full of therapy, bed rest, chiropractic adjustments, pills, heat, and cold packs, and a fair amount of depression. Everything helped, but nothing cured me. Then I read a book by a grateful patient of Dr. Alex Thompson. Dr. Thompson showed me how to adjust my own sacroiliac and he did Prolotherapy on me...I was one of the early ones.

The Prolotherapy and sacral adjustments helped stabilize me for years, until two years ago when a disc herniated. This time there was no relief. No physical therapy would help. An MRI showed a 12 mm bulge in the disc. My mindset was that I had an injury and a top surgeon told me that an operation was my only solution. My resolve against surgery weakened and so I scheduled the operation. But the week before, an old friend suggested that I consult with Marc Darrow, M.D.

The first day when I walked in bent over like a "C" was the beginning of magic. Dr. Darrow was not only reassuring, but almost presumptuous that he could cure me. My first treatment that day was with an MRA, a magnet resonance analyzer. The relief was so immediate that I went home and canceled the surgery. What followed was amazing. More MRA, then a wonderful form of chiropractic, then MedX, a back strengthening machine.

An MRI showed a 12 mm bulge in the disc.

To me, the MedX machine approached a miracle. I found that I gradually let go of the fixation of my disc protrusion causing my pain, and replaced it with a loving and healing optimism of the Joint Rehab group. Today I'm healed, my back is incredibly strong. I have gone from 70 pounds of resistance on the MedX to 180 pounds, and I haven't had a MedX treatment in a year. I maintained by doing yard work and going to the gym five days a week.

I guess what I've learned is this, that each doctor and therapist has his own bag of tricks, and if you go through it and they don't help, you should move on.

Believe you can be better. Let a positive mind work for you. Find the doctor and the staff that gives you energy. Most of all be open to new ideas. Be curious. Ask questions. Participate in your own care.

If your doctor doesn't interact, listen, or have time for you, change doctors. Today, alternative therapies are more visible and accessible than ever. Yesterday's mavericks are approaching mainstream. But, fortunately there will always be others. If you search, you will find your Joint Rehabilitation & Sports Medical Center, Inc., it's a wonderful way to experience your healing."

References

Ongley M, Klein R, Dorman T, Eek B, Hubert L. A new approach to the treatment of chronic low back pain. Lancet 1987;2:143-146.

Frymoyer JW. Back pain and sciatica. N Engl J Med 1988;318:291-300.

Hauser R, Hauser M. Prolo Your Sports Injuries Away! Jean-Paul Ouellette, M.D., (contributor.) Beulah Land Press, 2001:226.

McElligott J, Miscovich SJ, Fielding LP. Low back injury in industry: the value of a recovery program. Conn Med 1989;53:711-715.

Batti, MC, Bigos SJ. Industrial back pain complaints: a broader perspective. Orthop Clin North Am 1991;22:273-282.

Liebenson CS. Pathogenesis of chronic back pain. J Manipulative Physiol Ther 1992;15:299-308.

Andersson GB. Factors important in the genesis and prevention of occupational back pain and disability. J Manipulative Physiol Ther1992;15:43-46.

Gyntelberg F. One year incidence of low back pain among male residents of Copenhagen aged 40-59. Dan Med Bull 1974;21:30-36.

Frymoyer JW, Rosen JC, Clements J, et al. Psychologic factors in low-back-pain disability. Clin Orthop 1985;195: 178-184.

Pope MH, Rosen JC, Wilder DG, et al. The relation between biomechanical and psychological factors in patients with low-back pain. Spine 1980;5:173-178.

Marras W, Heaney C, Davis K, et al. Job stress may lead to back injury for some people, Spine December 2000.

Carragee E, Paragioudakis S, Khurana S. Stanford University Medical Center, State of mind contributes to low back pain, Spine December 2000.

Behrens V, Seligman P, Cameron L, et al. The prevalence of back pain, hand discomfort, and dermatitis in the US working population. Am J Public Health 1994;84:1780-1785.

Nelson B, Carpenter D. Can spinal surgery be prevented by aggressive strengthening exercises? A prospective study of cervical and lumbar patients. Archives of Physical Medicine and Rehabilitation 80 (Jan 1999): 20-25.

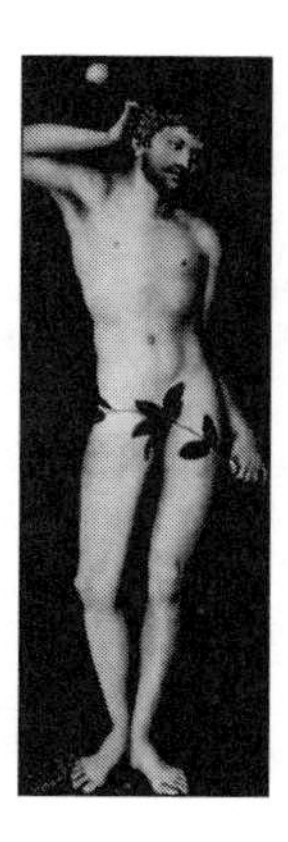

Chapter 7
Four Stories Of Knee Pain

When the doctor says: "I am recommending surgery, ultimately you will probably need a knee replacement because of the damage in there." There are two choices to make—one, accept your destiny and continue to live with an unstable and painful knee until the surgeon calls, or find a solution to your pain now.

Is Surgery the Ultimate Answer?

To someone wearing a knee brace, who regularly tapes ice on their knee and takes prescribed and over-the-counter pain medication, what else could there be but surgery?

The diagnosis of knee injury is, in my opinion, too dependant on many large machines and invasive techniques.

Your knee hurts so you visit the orthopedist. He uses his tools to figure out why your knee hurts. While some of these tools are very impressive, are they accurate?

Once x-rays rule out problems with bones, an MRI (Magnetic Resonance Imaging) is used because of its ability to reveal soft tissue damage. But problems with the knee, especially the cartilage, can still be very evasive and hard to pinpoint. Studies

have shown that the advanced technologies commonly used to diagnosis injuries are grievously insufficient to do the job.

In one study[1] conducted by Dr. J.A. Lawrance of Oxford, England, MRIs had a success rate of only 11% in diagnosing partial anterior cruciate ligament tears. In yet another study, focusing on the knee, doctors compared the findings of standard x-ray tests and physical examinations on 210 people—all of whom were self-described as pain free at the time of the testing. Although none of the participants exhibited any pain or other symptoms of pathology, and considered themselves completely healthy in regard to their knees, the test results yielded dramatic evidence of physical problems and abnormalities—including an incidence rate of 80% or better for arthritis, patellofemoral crepitus (grinding) in 94% of the women, high percentages of asymmetry and hypermobility, and a dozen other problems to varying degrees. As the authors of the study noted:

> ***"Because patellofemoral crepitus is so common in both symptomatic and asymptomatic volunteers, the importance of this finding must be reevaluated as a surgical indication."***

The conclusion is obvious: By offering "objective" evidence and a technology-based rationale to surgeons, MRIs, x-rays and other advanced diagnostic techniques contribute greatly to promoting cases of unnecessary or even ill-advised surgery. The end result is more problems for the recipients of these surgeries.

Generally speaking, the most efficient and safe method for diagnosing a knee injury is a simple manual examination, coupled with extensive questioning of the patient to determine exactly what happened and where it hurts.

"Arthritis Surgery In Ailing Knees Cited As Sham"

"Common Knee Surgery Doesn't Relieve Arthritis"

"Study Finds Common Knee Surgery No Better Than Placebo"

Those were some of the headlines that made the news. What inspired them was one study and two editorials published in the July 11, 2002 issue of the New England Journal of Medicine which debated whether arthroscopic surgery for arthritis was effective or not. The debate was decidedly one-sided as the above headlines indicated.[2-4]

To make a long study short, the Department of Veteran's Affairs (VA) and Baylor College of Medicine researchers took 180 subjects who suffered from knee pain and divided them into three groups. The first group had surgical debridement performed, the procedure where bad cartilage is removed by cutting it away and removing it with an arthroscope. A second group underwent arthroscopic lavage, in which the knee is flushed out with a saline solution. The third group had a placebo surgery. Small incisions were made in the skin on the knee but no actual surgery was performed.

In the follow-up, patients were surveyed for two years following their real or placebo procedure. In some instances the placebo group reported better results!

> ***Researchers noted that it appeared the surgical procedure was worthless.***

It's in Your Knee For a Reason

Removing tissue from your knee can only make your knee weaker in the long run and prone to arthritis. This is why many have numerous surgeries on their knees, trying to correct problems in part caused by tissue removal.

Removal of the meniscus (or knee cartilage) decreases the shock absorption that protects the knee. Why shave it then? Because some physicians believe that the meniscus does not have the ability to be repaired, either by regular body repair mechanisms or surgery. So it is shaved, smoothed, or partially removed. Years ago, when a meniscus was injured, the standard protocol was complete

removal and resultant bone-on-bone arthritis in the future. Many of these poor patients were forced to have knee replacements years later because of the severe pain from the meniscus removal.

Removing knee tissue can never make the knee as strong as it once was.

Your tendons, ligaments, cartilage and meniscus, are all in your knee for a reason. They serve a purpose. Removing or cutting any of the tissue makes your knee weaker and more prone to arthritis.

The Tools Of Arthroscopy

The tool used in arthroscopy is the arthroscope, a 14-inch-long metal tube, which is as thick as a woman's finger. It is inserted deep into the joint, allowing the physician to see inside the knee for a close-up look at the problem. What allows the surgeon to see so well is that the knee is inflated with water, forcing the bones to be pushed apart to allow the intruder the room it needs to see, shave, cut, and drill into the tissues that hold your knee together, without large incisions (open procedure). The reason why arthroscopy is so popular in sports medicine is that it is less evasive and heals sooner so the athlete can return to play sooner.

Of course stretching out the tendons and ligaments and blowing up the knee capsule for easier surgical maneuvers may negatively impact the natural structure and in the long-term lead to arthritis.

Why Every Part of the Knee is Important

To understand the theory (and folly) of this seemingly harmless procedure, one needs to understand the physiological composition of the joint. Most of the joints in the body are synovial joints, which means they are flexible and self-lubricating. The ends of the bones are covered with a protective substance known as articular cartilage. These thin coatings are separated by a layer of

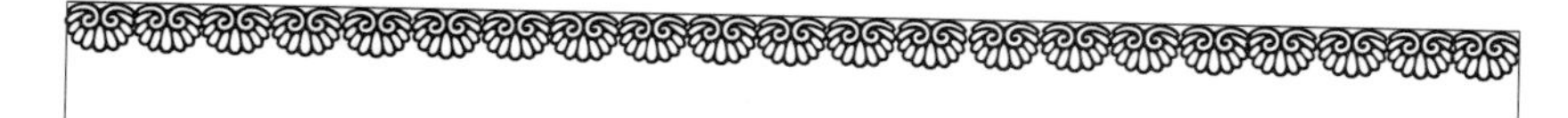

synovial fluid, which further cushions and lubricates them where they meet to form the joint.

Ligaments add support and hold the joints together. Tendons secure the muscles, which provide movement to the body. The whole structure is wrapped in a collagen capsule and synovial membrane, which also secretes the lubricating and somewhat revitalizing synovial fluid.

The knee also contains pads of fibrous cartilage, known as menisci, which help these overworked joints bear the extra stresses to which they are often subjected.

The articular cartilage which provides a smooth surface for the bones to slide on each other in the joint, is a homogenous substance devoid of nerves, lymphatic vessels or blood cells, it is made up primarily of water, collagen and specialized proteins (proteoglycans). Its structure is fairly simple; it contains a small percentage of cells known as chondrocytes, which are solely responsible for the maintenance and repair of the articular cartilage, via their ability to synthesize collagen and proteoglycans.

The high water content of the articular cartilage, coupled with the innate compressibility of the proteoglycans, give it the slick, cushioning properties so essential to maintaining healthy, pain free joints, minimizing friction and stress between the bones.

All the available evidence seems to indicate that chondrocytes are fully capable of regenerating articular cartilage throughout the course of a lifetime, which would account for the healthy cell counts even in very old people. However, since they are not fed by blood vessels, they are wholly dependent on nutrient delivery from the synovial fluid; this lack of blood supply puts a damper on their proliferative capabilities.

It is the movement of the joints that loads nutrients into, and waste out of, the cartilage. Despite their limited metabolic resources, chondrocytes can still churn out large quantities of collagen and proteoglycans.

The invasive tools of arthroscopic surgery are used to excise injured ligaments, tendons, cartilage and meniscus, which leads to a further depletion of the articular cartilage (because the

meniscus supplies nutrients to it)—either through shaving or slicing with a high-powered electrical instrument.

The immediate result may be a respite from whatever pain existed before the procedure, but is often followed by permanent weakness and instability in the joint and resultant pain in years to come.

Unfortunately, such "collateral damage" seems more acceptable to the industrialized medical establishment than less invasive (and less profit-oriented) therapies like trigger point injections and Prolotherapy. It would be somewhat comforting to know that such intensely destructive surgical procedures are falling from favor, if it weren't for the fact that other, less obvious, but equally damaging techniques, such as NSAIDs and anti-inflammatory medications, are still wide-spread.

The damage NSAIDs and anti-inflammatory medications do is permanent and extensive. Effective at reducing pain because of their anti-inflammatory action, cortisone and other Corticosteroids can assault the body with an avalanche of counter-productive side effects if used repeatedly.

Even worse, although exercise normally strengthens the body, studies have shown that when cortisone is injected into the knees, and the patient exercises, there is even greater destruction than with cortisone shots alone, with cartilage cell counts reduced by over 20%.

Steroids inhibit the release of growth hormone and rob the body of calcium and vitamin D. They also interfere with the development of new tissue growth and disrupt the processes that lead to new cell and blood vessel formation.

Corticosteroids inhibit the synthesis of proteins, collagen, and proteoglycans in articular cartilage by inhibiting chondrocyte production, the cells that comprise and produce the articular cartilage.

The net catabolic effect (chemical decomposition) of repeated corticosteroids is inhibition of fibroblast production of collagen, ground substance, and angiogenesis (new blood vessel formation). The result is weakened synovial joints, supporting structures, articular cartilage, ligaments, and tendons. This weakness increases the pain, and the increased pain leads to more steroid injections.

A study by Dr. Behrens[5] and his colleagues reported a persistent and highly significant reduction in the synthesis of proteins, collagen, and proteoglycans in the articular cartilage of rabbits who received weekly injections of glucocorticoids. They also reported a progressive loss of endoplasmic reticulum, mitochondria, and Golgi apparatus, as the number of injections increased.

Trigger point injections and Prolotherapy offer a radically different approach than either arthroscopic or corticosteroidal therapy.

The two latter methods often yield temporary relief with their "quick fix" procedures—but may be followed by highly destructive long-term side effects including irreversible damage.

By contrast, trigger point injections and Prolotherapy deliver permanent improvement, including not only pain relief but strengthening of the treated areas.

The Complexity of the Knee

The patella, commonly called the kneecap, sits in a groove at the front of the knee. The most common knee problems encountered in clinical practice involve the patella, because its anatomical

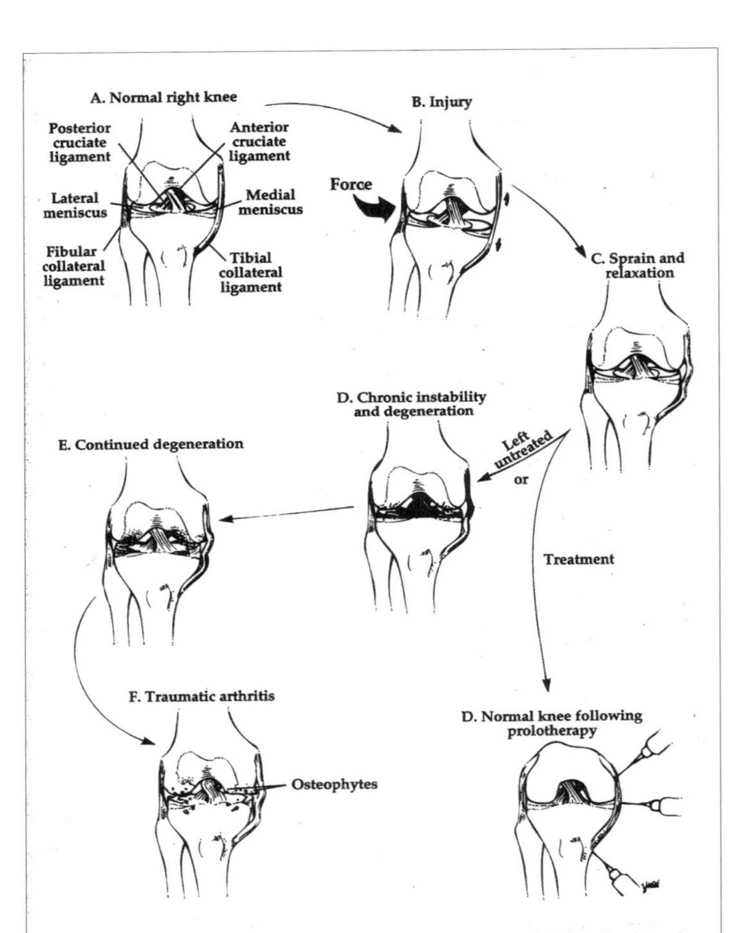

Fig. 8.6 Following trauma, the ligaments become sprained. When healing does not occur, the ligaments become relaxed, resulting in chronic instability and degeneration. When left untreated, post-traumatic "arthritis" or degenerative osteoarthritis follows. This degenerative process can be prevented with appropriate intervention through prolotherapy.

placement subjects it directly to a variety of bone and soft tissue disorders.

A portion of the general population is subject to these disorders, which include:

Patellofemoral syndrome (patella mistracks in femoral groove);

Excessive torsional deformity of the tibia;

High or lateral position of the patella;

Shallow femoral trochlea;

Atrophy of vastus medialus oblique muscle;

Increased quadriceps angle (often in those with wide hips);

Over-development of the vastus lateralis muscles;

Flat feet;

Excessive pronation of the feet (feet turn up to the side).

Behind the patella is a layer of articular cartilage—the thickest layer of cartilage found in any of the joints of the body.

Until recently, we did not know that cartilage is directly treatable by trigger point injections and Prolotherapy. We knew the benefits Prolotherapy offered in adjoining soft tissue, due to the strengthening of the supporting ligaments and tendons, which keep the joints properly aligned and thereby protect the cartilage from erosion caused by friction.

A recent study, showed that Prolotherapy stimulates the growth of articulate cartilage[6].

In this study, people who had knee arthritis, and, who suffered from knee pain for an average of eight years or more, received Prolotherapy over a six month period. Important to note is that 35% of the knees examined for the study had no cartilage remaining in one or more major compartments.

The results? Thirty-five percent (35%) reduction of pain, 45% improvement in swelling and 67% improvement in knee buckling as well as a 13 degree improvement in knee range of motion.

Prolotherapy works on most knee problems with excellent results. Only in the case of a completely torn ligament is Prolotherapy somewhat limited. If there is a partial tear (sometimes on MRI these may look like complete tears) Prolotherapy may be able to reconstruct the ligament and strengthen the joint. But even with a complete tear, Prolotherapy is extremely beneficial because an impact with enough force to completely rupture a ligament will also loosen the entire knee structure. Prolotherapy in this situation can strengthen the surrounding tissues giving the patient a better chance of long-term success.

It is rare that a patient who is not active in sports or a competitive athlete needs ACL surgery. Many athletes function on an ACL deficient knee.

Surgery

There are certainly instances in life when surgery is called for, but not nearly as often as it is currently performed. Even so-called "minor" surgery takes a drastic toll on the human body, physically traumatizing and permanently altering its structures, often to its detriment.

Ernie Banks, Baseball Immortal

Sports fans will know that the following patient's story comes from one of the true gentlemen in sports. Known for five decades as "Mr. Cub," Ernie Banks was a forerunner of today's modern baseball shortstop. Big, strong, a powerful home run hitter and graceful fielder.

Ernie knows that many people remember him in his days as one of baseball's most feared hitters and that the sight of him limping around could be very disconcerting to a lot of his fans.

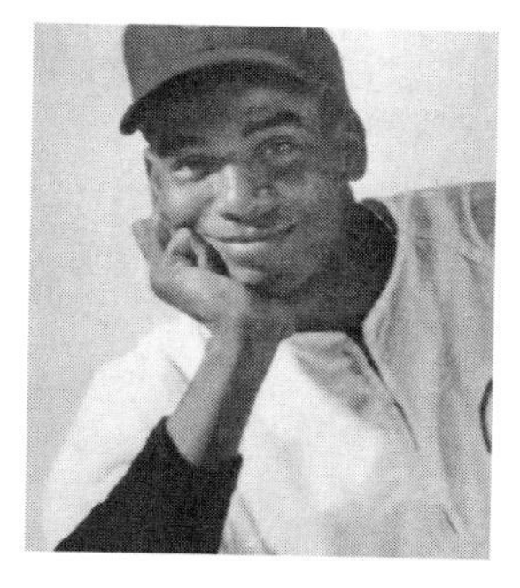

Ernie Banks

"The one unusual thing about playing professional baseball is that when you retire, and people see you limping around, it bothers them. They call my wife and say *'What in the world is wrong with Ernie? Do something. He can't even walk. We remember him running.'*"

As Ernie reached his mid-50's, his knee pain really began to escalate.

"The pain became more severe when I was 55. I retired from baseball when I was 40 but still played in Old-Timer's games until I was 50. Finally I had to stop because of stiffness (in the knees) and a little more pain.

Many doctors told me that I would need total knee replacements, like many of my friends have had. But I never had them. I felt that type of surgery wouldn't help me at all in terms of my sports life."

Ernie has arthritic knees, and like many, he took it for granted that an active man who reaches his 60's and 70's was simply destined to have severe arthritis.

"My knees were arthritic and I couldn't walk well, I couldn't run, and at night they were very painful.

Then I came to my real good friend, Dr. Darrow. He says to me, 'Let's try this, let's do that.' I was a little hesitant because my greatest fear is needles, but Marc convinced me to get Prolotherapy. So I did.

Prolotherapy has given me more flexibility, in my legs and my knees. I can work out and I use a lot of heavy weight programs to build up the quadriceps. My whole body is feeling better and I just feel that one of these days I will feel good enough to play another season of baseball."

Sally Kirkland

Sally Kirkland is an Oscar Nominee and Golden Globe Winner for **Anna**, a veteran of over 70 films including Ron Howard's film **ED T.V.** in which she played Ed's mom and appeared as "Anita Mann," in the Jim Carrey comedy "Bruce Almighty."

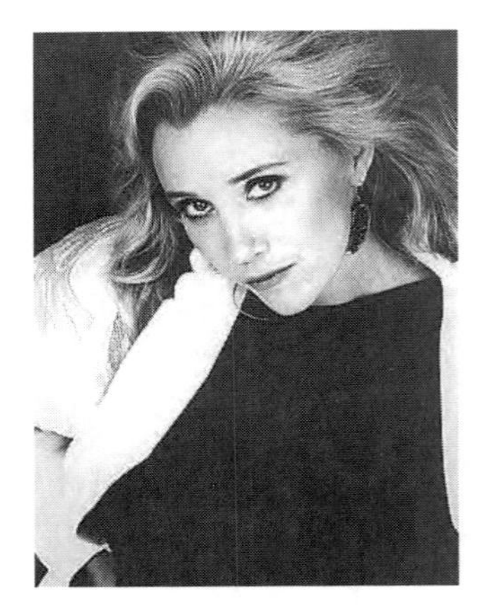

Sally Kirkland

She writes about her experiences with knee pain and its healing at ***Joint Rehabilitation***.

"I want to write a testimony to a health center called the Joint Rehabilitation Center. I have been in the theater, film, and TV industry since the 1960's. It can be very stressful to say the least. I have always taken a stand for alternative health as my 100 percent survival mode for working grueling hours in sometimes unhealthy conditions.

I have spoken out worldwide about silicon toxicity and the crippling effects my silicone implants left me with for ten years. My silicone, then saline implants, were explanted by 1998. I had massive rupturing of silicone implants, the toxicity settled in my joints and muscles and organs. It has been one of the biggest challenges in my life. At Joint Rehabilitation and Sports Medical Center, I met with Dr. Jason Kelberman who has been working with me on two accounts. One, as before mentioned, and two, a broken foot and injured knee and leg I've had since a car accident in April, 2000.

Jason Kelberman has been using a technique on me called Applied Kinesiology, the study of movement of the body. He worked with what he calls muscle dysfunction and gait abnormality. He is an extraordinary chiropractor.

The next miracle was Dr. Marc Darrow and something called Prolotherapy. When I had the accident with my foot and knee, the foot responded well to chiropractic but the knee had such excruciating pain. I interviewed with doctors on three different kinds of knee surgeries. I had a very tough time sleeping with the pain. I was able to sleep only a few hours per night and in between the pain. I began to talk to friends who had had knee replacement surgery. Then, a friend suggested I see Marc Darrow, M.D.

He told me about his work with Prolotherapy and how the injections would not just block the pain but rebuild the collagen. I had never heard of such a thing. He anesthetized the knee and then gave me a series of Prolo injections.

It was a total miracle to me. I was not yet at 100 percent, but enough to be able to function, to get some sleep, and drive without spasms.

I agreed to have more injections over a period of months and I called off the surgery.

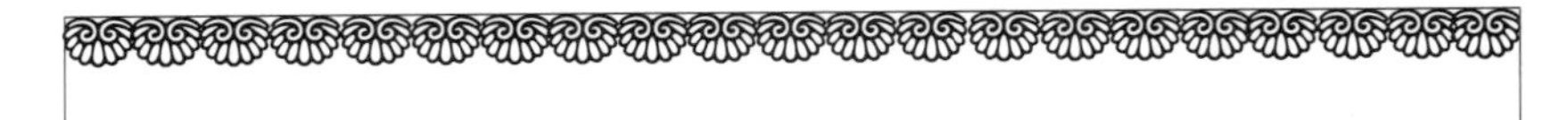

I feel like Dr. Darrow has given me back my knee, and he and Dr. Kelberman gave me back my foot.

Now, my physical strength is on its way back. Dr. Darrow and Dr. Kelberman have been inspiring me to cut any and all acidic foods and liquids from my nutritional sensibility. Obviously, no caffeine, no sugar and no dairy. They can all apparently irritate injuries and joint and muscle pain.

Dr. Kelberman is one of the best spinal adjusters I've ever worked with. He has done cranial sacral balancing and upper cervical adjustments with me. He has also been working with me to balance emotional exhaustion connected to the physical pain and sleep deprivation. Dr. Darrow and Kelberman then sent me to their Ph.D. exercise physiologist, Dr. Bill Bergman. I feel like I have known him 30 years. I have worked with strengthening my foot, legs, back, upper arms, and torso, all in the safest conditions I've ever experienced."

Abdul-Karim Al-Jabbar, NFL Running Back

In 1996, the Miami Dolphins used their third round pick in the National Football League's annual college draft to take a running back out of the University of California at Los Angeles named Karim Abdul-Jabbar (now Abdul-Karim Al-Jabbar.)

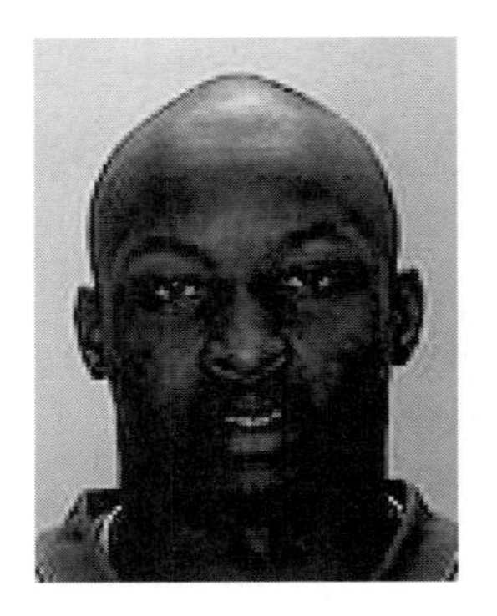

Abdul-Karim Al-Jabbar

Karim may have slipped down to the third round because a player with a history of knee problems would tend to scare off some professional teams, but Karim had talent and the desire that made him appealing to many clubs and he wound up a Miami Dolphin.

In 1993, at UCLA, Karim began to experience the knee

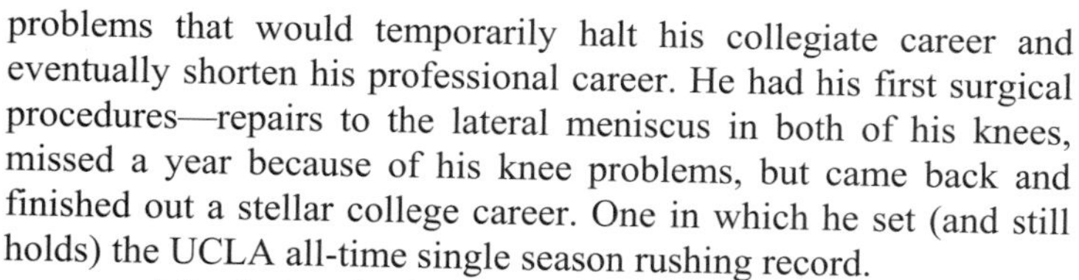

problems that would temporarily halt his collegiate career and eventually shorten his professional career. He had his first surgical procedures—repairs to the lateral meniscus in both of his knees, missed a year because of his knee problems, but came back and finished out a stellar college career. One in which he set (and still holds) the UCLA all-time single season rushing record.

After being drafted by the Dolphins, Karim paid off the team's confidence in him by becoming the first player in that franchise's storied history to rush for over 100 yards in his first NFL game. Later that season, Karim became the first Dolphin in 20 years to top the 1,000 yard mark in rushing, all while working out of the backfield with the all-time NFL great Dan Marino.

To prove that his rookie year was no fluke, the next year, (1997) Karim lead the NFL in touchdowns.

The future was as bright as it could be until Karim's knee problems worsened. By 2001, the brightness had faded and Karim's career was over.

"It was my right knee. I had a total of four surgeries, the last after my career ended in 2001 where they went in there to clean up the meniscus.

> ***My biggest problem with my knee was the swelling. I could never heal or rehab properly because of it. I did do all the proper rehab and followed the proper nutrition, but my knee would still swell. I could never get to rehab it to the level that I wanted to."***

After all the surgical procedures, Karim was left with a chronically swollen knee, pain, and a loss of mobility. Then some strange things started happening.

"A friend handed me a copy of (Dr. Darrow's book), The Collagen Revolution, Living Pain Free. She thought it was what I needed so I gave Dr. Darrow a call.

I know my knee was a mess, but after the first Prolotherapy injection, it was like a miracle. I had swelling in my knee for ten years, (and within a week) it was gone and hasn't returned."

Not only had the swelling gone down, but Karim's activity level increased dramatically.

"It was a blessing. I can play with my kids now. I played racquetball for the first time, and I couldn't even dream about doing something like that (with the condition of my knees.)"

Karim's knees felt so good that he took on a challenge that would rival any extreme sport or training challenge.

"You know I promised myself once that I would run the dunes at Manhattan Beach ten times. If I could do it, it would convince me that I had NFL talent, for some reason I never got the chance to run the dunes. Now these sand dunes are very high, maybe at a 60 degree angle. Every step is like taking four. After the Prolotherapy I ran the dunes for the first time!"

Maybe Karim was convincing himself that he would be an NFL talent again!

"My knee got better really fast! It was amazing! Obviously if I would have known about Prolotherapy before all the surgeries I definitely would have went in and got the injections. Just not having all the swelling would have changed my career!"

Karim is a young man of 29 with the mentality of an elite athlete. Is his career really over?

"I haven't written off football. You still have to get strong and do things to get back onto the field (to play at that level.)"

To Tell The Truth, Prolotherapy Worked

Orson Bean is a veteran of over 50 years in television, younger fans remember him as Loren Bray from "Dr. Quinn Medicine Woman" and Bill Gamble on "Normal, Ohio." Orson has also been a guest star on "7th Heaven", "Will & Grace", "The King of

Queens", and "Ally McBeal". In the movies, he was nominated for a Screen Actors Guild Award in 2000 for "Being John Malkovich."

Many of us also remember Orson for his years on "To Tell The Truth", "Matchgame", "Password", a classic role on the legendary "The Twilight Zone," and for his 200 or so appearances on the "Tonight Show with Johnny Carson" as a guest and guest host.

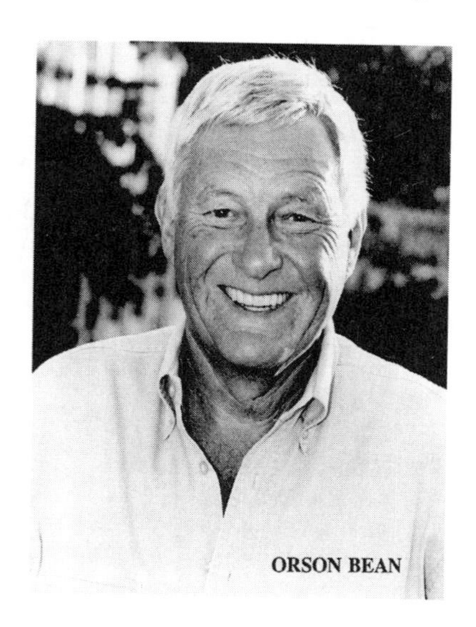
ORSON BEAN

Ironically enough Orson's knee problems began on the set of "Dr. Quinn Medicine Woman," a show about a pioneer woman physician.

"In the course of this show I had to play a role in which I broke my leg. I hopped around on one foot for a week on steep mountainsides and really banged the hell out of my knee. It did not get better, so I went to see a doctor who advised me to have arthroscopic surgery.

He said it should last you 10 years and then you are going to be looking at a knee replacement.

Well, he was right. It did last 10 years, then, it began hurting again. I went back to him and he said, like I told you, knee replacement.

So, in desperation, I went to see the crazy guy I heard about on the radio, Marc Darrow, and said well, what can I lose? It was three shots later the knee felt fine, and that has been almost a year and a half, and I have had no pain whatsoever."

The 76-year old actor has no time to be slowed down by knee pain, at the time of this writing, Orson was preparing to star in a revival of the classic musical "Brigadoon."

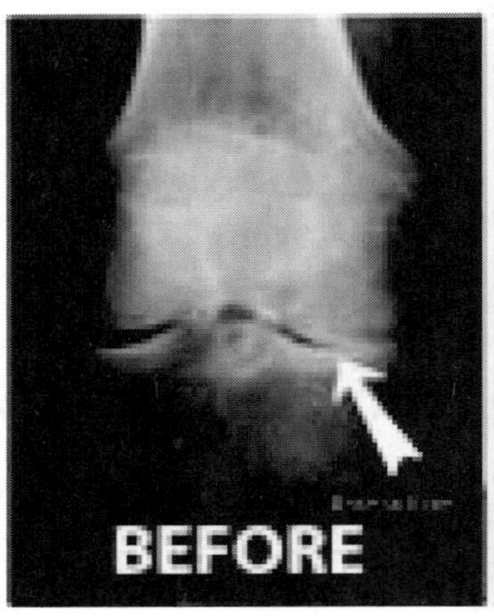

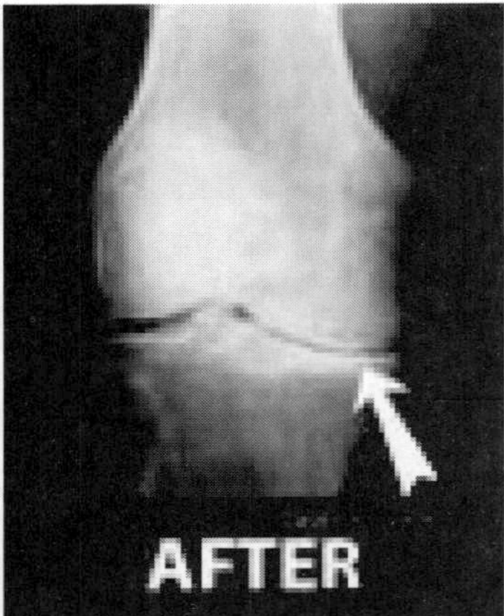

From his book, ***Prolotherapy, An Alternative to Knee Surgery*** (www.beulahlandpress.com) my colleague Ross Hauser, M.D., of Oak Park, Illinois shows a patient's x-ray. The before picture shows bone-on-bone. The after picture shows regeneration of cartilage after Prolotherapy.

References

Behrens F, Shepard N, Mitchell N. Alterations of rabbit articular cartilage by intra-articular injections of glucocorticoids. J Bone Joint Surg (Am) 1975;57(1):70-6

Lui YK. et al. An in situ study of the influence of a sclerosing solution in rabbit medial collateral ligaments and its junction strength. Connective Tissue Research, 1983;11:95-102.

Hackett GA, Henderson DG. Joint stabilization: an experimental, histologic study with comments on the clinical application in ligament proliferation. American Journal of Surgery, 1955;89:968-973.

Reeves KD Hassanein K Randomized prospective double-blind placebo-controlled study of dextrose prolotherapy for knee osteo arthritis with or without ACL laxity. Alt Ther Hlth Med 2000;6(2):37-46.

Dorman T. Prolotherapy for Knees. Townsend Letter for Doctors and Patients, November, 1997.

Lawrance JA, et al. MRI diagnosis of partial tears of the anterior cruciate ligament. Injury, 1996;27;3:153-155.

Johnson L. Clinical assessment of asymptomatic knees. Arthroscopy, 1998;14:347-359.

Neumann RD. Sports Medicine Secrets. Hanley & Belfus, Inc., 1994;66:291.

Van Pelt R, (contributor). Prolo Your Sports Injury Away, Hauser R, Hauser M, (editors). Beulah Land Press, 2001,p.272.

Mankin H. The Articular Cartilage: A Review. American Academy of Orthopedic Surgeons: Instructional Course Lectures. C.V. Mosby, St. Louis, 1970;19.

Scott W. Dr. Scott's Knee Book. Fireside Press, New York. 1996, p.36.

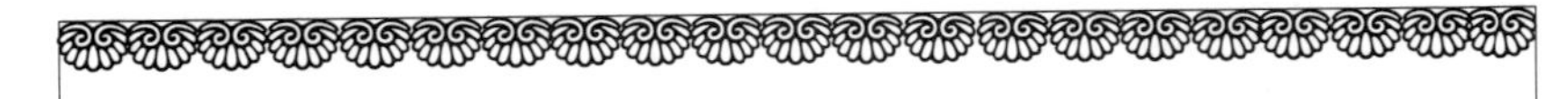

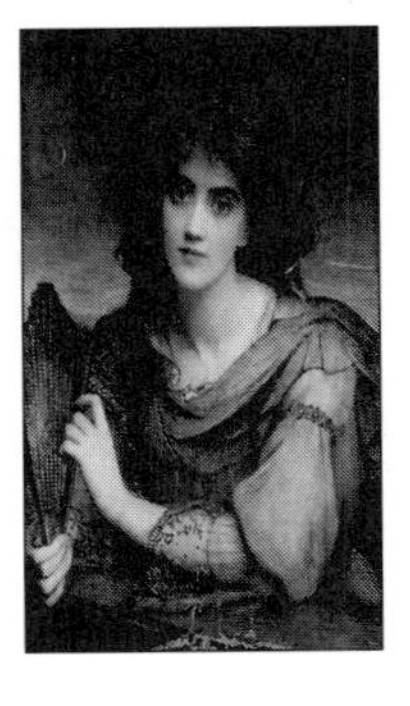

"Resolve to be happy, and your joy shall form and invincible host against difficulty"
—Helen Keller—

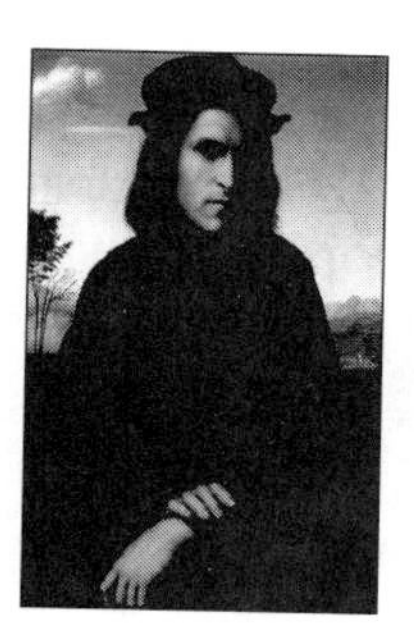

Chapter 8
Prolotherapy for Hand, Wrist and Elbow Injuries

If you recall my own story in chapter one, you know that I suffered terribly from "tennis elbow." I was told by doctors that I just had to learn to live with the pain. I did because all I knew was traditional remedies which did not work for me. Steroid injections reduced the pain temporarily, but the pain just got worse.

When I later learned about Prolotherapy, I used it to strengthen the ligaments and tendons that held my elbow together. Once the area was strengthened, the muscle pain also disappeared because the muscles did not have to continue to overcompensate. The ligament and tendon pain disappeared because new collagen grew and rejuvenated my elbow.

The Culprits of Chronic Elbow and Wrist Pain

The annular ligament connects and stabilizes the two bones of the forearm, the ulna and the radius. Activities that involve rotation of the elbow, such as screwing in a light bulb, turning a screw driver, or using a cork screw, put a tremendous stress on this ligament. It especially includes those activities in sports where throwing is involved, or where a club is used to drive a ball. Pain

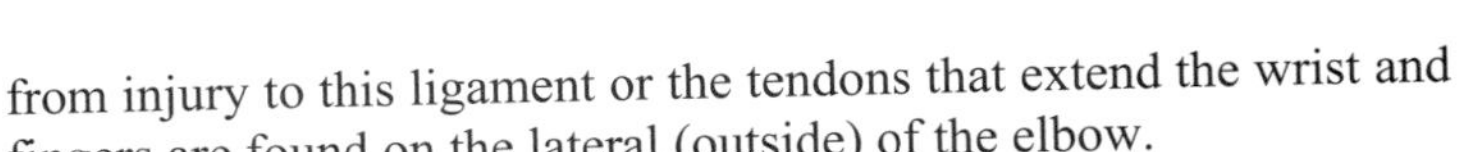

from injury to this ligament or the tendons that extend the wrist and fingers are found on the lateral (outside) of the elbow.

While an acute injury, like a fall, can be responsible for an annular ligament or extensor tendon injury, it is usually repetitive motion that does it. This type of elbow injury can last for months or years and is usually diagnosed under the umbrella term "Tennis Elbow."

Sometimes the pain in the annular ligament can refer down into the thumb, wrist, and index and middle fingers, mimicking and sometimes leading to an incorrect diagnosis of Carpal Tunnel Syndrome.

"Golfer's Elbow" is another umbrella term coined to describe elbow pain when flexing the wrist and hand as in activities of grasping, clutching, and typing. It gets its name "Golfer's Elbow" because the muscles and tendons required to hit a golf ball are the same ones used in these flexion activities.

The ligament involved in Golfer's Elbow is the ulnar collateral ligament (UCL) which holds the ulnar bone of the forearm to the bottom of the upper arm bone (the humerus.) When this ligament is injured or weakened, its pain can be felt on the medial side (inside) of the elbow.

Once determined that it is weakness or injury to the tendons or ligament that is causing elbow pain, Prolotherapy can be administered and the pain can be resolved.

Chronic Pain in Hand, Wrist and Elbow for a Long Drive Champion and Fitness Inventor Lee Brandon, CNCS.

"That CNCS (Certified strength and conditioning specialist) after my name, I worked hard for that," says Lee. "I've been a certified strength and conditioning specialist for many years. I worked with the 1984 Olympic team, I was the head strength and conditioning specialist for the nationally ranked softball team at Delphi University, I worked for Hofstra University as an adjunct professor for six years, and as their head strength and conditioning coach for seven years, running 14 of their teams in their women's programs."

One thing Lee knows is strength and fitness, so when a wrist injury failed to heal, she sought out a treatment that would give her the best chance of healing.

"Prolotherapy for me was a miracle because I had so much pain. I am not into surgery and wanted to give my body every chance to heal naturally and on its own."

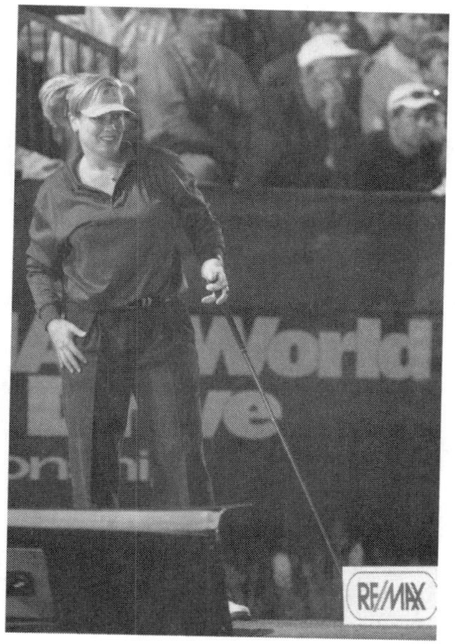

Lee Brandon
Photo by Ed Dosien

Lee has an incredible story to tell that goes back to a tragic accident. In 1979 Lee had to have her left arm partially reattached after she fell through a window. The injury ended a promising career, one geared towards competing in the 1980 Olympics.

Prior to the injury Lee was a nationally ranked shot putter, discus thrower and softball player. "I still hold the softball throw record (209 feet) in my junior high school. I had 'an arm on me'. I was always a gifted athlete, yet it took me seven years to use my arm again."

After the accident Lee began a new career. "In the last 10 years I have been running two separate companies.

One is an intellectual properties company, I am the inventor of AB-vanced Neu-Spine Technologies®. Injuries, as we get older are inevitable, AB-vanced Neu-Spine Technologies® is a

whole school of movement where I simply state posture equals power. I'm a firm believer that ultimately, if one knows how to stabilize core and postural muscles, where your brain actually helps stabilize the spine, that you can re-coordinate your body and retrain your body to do correct strength training, correct flexibility problems, and correctly do cardiovascular training in a very symmetrical and balanced format. I believe ultimately you can greatly enhance your ability to avoid injury."

The Rise To Long-Drive Champion

Following her successes in the fitness business, Lee returned to competition-by accident. "I got into golf by default. It was one of my clients who brought me to a driving range. He had a bit of a spine issue so he stuck his driver in my hand and said, 'well, show me (the right way to swing.')

I had never hit a golf ball before, it had been years since I even swung at a softball because of my accident. So I took a field hockey slap at it and it went like 250 yards!

My client looked at me and said: 'keep the stupid driver, I don't want it anymore!'

It was actually pretty funny. But he saw golfing talent in me and bought me my first lesson with a golf professional.

"Now I am hitting them even farther"

I enjoyed the game and played a little on and off but I was way too busy running my companies, training clients at the gym and doing a lot of corporate fitness training classes."

Yet Lee's competitive nature lead her to re-enter the field of competition and in October 2001 she won the Remax® World Long Drive Championship with a drive of 291 yards.

To Lee that drive is not nearly as impressive as the ones she is hitting today. "Now I am hitting them even farther," she says.

Prolotherapy Enhances Lee's Long Drive Golf Game

As much as we would like to say Prolotherapy helped Lee to the championship, it did not. Lee won the Long Drive Championship despite a severe hand injury and before she began Prolotherapy treatments.

We can say, however, that since she started Prolotherapy she is hitting the ball better. "I'm consistently hitting 15 to 35 yards further this year then last year, and without the pain I once had."

Injured Before the Championship

"About three weeks before the championship I damaged my left hand. The tendons in that hand are very much at risk because of the rigidity due to the injury where the scar is located. I was trying out a couple of new drivers when I hit the dirt too hard and severely sprained the tendon in my left hand.

"But I competed, basically one-handed, and won the championship. It was just a pure miracle that I was able to walk away winning.

"Two months later I was still in a lot of pain, I thought the injury would heal by itself but it didn't. When I came to see you (Dr. Darrow) in December of 2001 my left wrist was very painful, as well as my right elbow. I had tendinitis in my right arm because it was taking so much of the heat of my left one not working. That had actually been going on for a year-and-a-half. The left wrist that I injured before the championship was now in its third month of chronic pain.

"While my right wrist was never a problem, I was concerned that it was handling a lot of the load that my left wrist couldn't so I had Prolotherapy done on it. It was more for prevention.

"Three weeks following the first treatment I started noticing a difference. The pain went away and as a matter of fact my grip is stronger.

"I'm weight training again with the heavy stuff! I lift 225 pounds, I squat 225, I mean I'm doing some exciting things for my age with perfect form. My bone density was just tested. I'm at 117%!

"After this I would tell anyone who asked, don't hesitate to get Prolotherapy! Find a doctor like Dr. Darrow who performs it in a very strategic personalized way so that you have it done exactly right."

A Producer's Chronic Elbow Pain

Making a motion picture requires a lot of behind the scenes people. While the general notion that the stars make a picture a success or lack of stars make the picture a failure, a film will never get to this stage without the Hollywood producer.

Producers are aptly named because they do just that, produce movies. One of the ways they produce movies is to broker the deals necessary to ensure the multi-million dollar funding the picture needs to get off the ground.

I was experiencing horrendous pain.

One such producer is Bernie Williams, "(Back in) 1999 I had a lot of pain in my right elbow. I can joke now that I probably got it from writing out those huge checks for the movies I make. Seriously though, I was experiencing horrendous pain for over six months."

Bernie has been in the business a long time, his resume includes producing such films as "Dirty Rotten Scoundrels" with Michael Caine and Steve Martin, "What About Bob?" with Bill Murray and Richard Dreyfuss, "Who's That Girl?" with Madonna, "Ragtime", the last movie of the great James Cagney, "Mutiny on the Bounty" with Mel Gibson, and "Daredevil" with Ben Affleck.

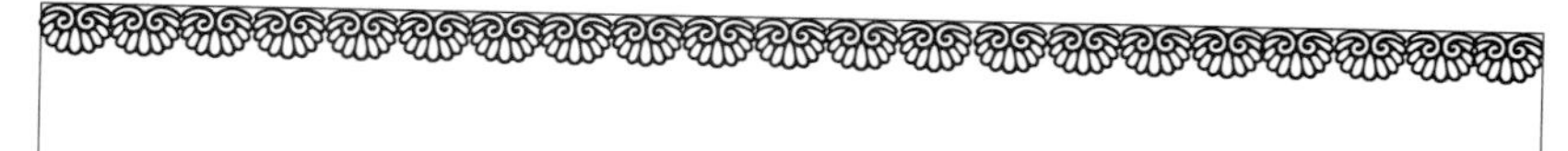

Writing the big checks is not what caused Bernie's pain, but rather a more humanitarian activity. "When I am not financing movies, I help run a 'non-kill' dog shelter.

"Some of the dogs we have are big, real big. When they are leashed they really pull on my arms, especially my right arm. Once the pain in my elbow started, it got really bad. Some people call this pain, tennis elbow. I call it ***'over-active dog elbow.'***

"I had great reservations about Prolotherapy, being a little skeptical—and I hate injections anyway," Bernie says, but once he got those injections, his reservations were lost.

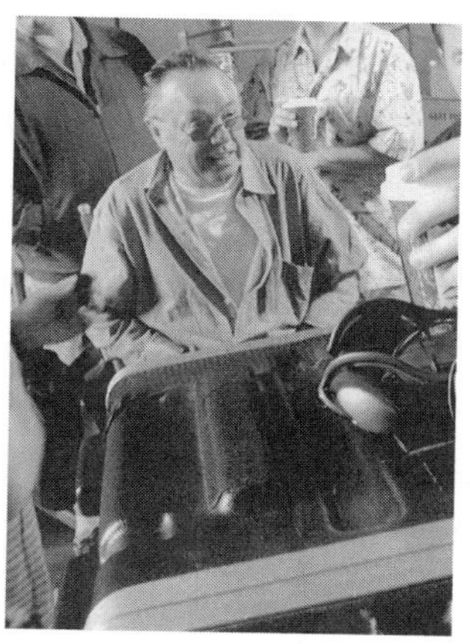

Bernie Williams

"I came here to Joint Rehab a few times and had those few shots with you and I gotta tell you, within a matter of weeks it (the pain) disappeared and it has not returned.

I'm still working with the dogs. Still picking up dog crates and having big dogs take me for a walk. My right arm is now my strength arm. Being able to work with these dogs is my way of giving back to society for the great life I have. It is also very rewarding and helps center me. It makes me realize that these animals, which are not just dogs, all animals depend on us, and how much society is cruel to animals generally, especially dogs, because they're your best friends. And, they are very forgiving and loving." Bernie adds, "And I'm still writing checks for movies."

Another Case of Tennis Elbow: Mike Torchia

"I was learning how to play tennis when I got tennis elbow. I wasn't using proper technique, I was muscling the ball and my elbow took all the pressure. My elbow got so bad that I couldn't even lean on it.

Because Marc (Dr. Darrow) personally had tennis elbow and shoulder problems I knew he would know what to do."

Usually it takes a few treatments over a few weeks to strengthen the elbow joint enough to alleviate pain, but in Mike's case, it just took one treatment. "It was one incredible treatment! Initially I was expecting the Prolotherapy to take a while to work, a few months, maybe longer.

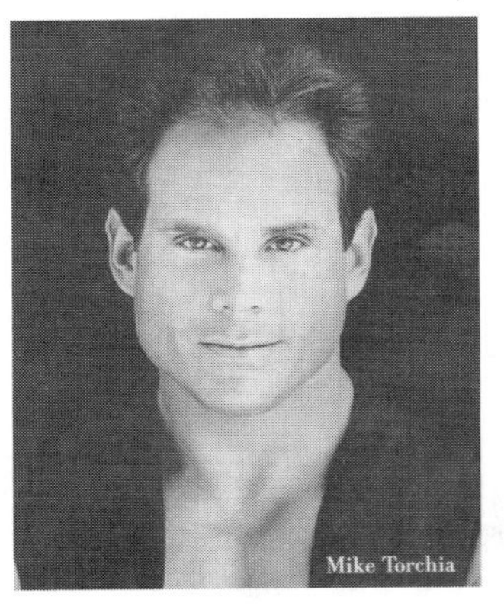

Mike Torchia

"But after the one treatment, the pain was gone (and hasn't come back.)"

So great was Mike's pain relief in his elbow that when his shoulder acted up, he was back for more injections.

"I was in New York for a photo shoot for this European magazine. They wanted a shot of me using the scapula chest machine. It was kind of drafty in the fitness center, I wasn't warmed up, so when I did the whole stack (of weights) for the shot, it strained the tendon and the ligaments in my shoulder. We (Dr. Darrow and I) did one session, a series of shots in the key point areas.

"I'd say within three weeks it started feeling incredibly better. Within two months it was like nothing ever happened. I responded every time you've given me Prolotherapy.

"I followed your instructions, resting, and so on, how to properly train while it was repairing, and it has worked fine, without anti-inflammatories, perfectly.

"I think Prolotherapy is sensational. I think that it's a method that is going to really open more opportunity for people to heal correctly, an opportunity for people to actually experience how to get healthy without using massive drugs to mask the pain."

Elbow Pain or Carpal Tunnel Syndrome?

Carpal Tunnel Syndrome is a compression of the median nerve at the wrist, leading to numbness tingling and pain in the hand. The median nerve passes through the carpal tunnel at the wrist and into the palm where it sends branches that control feeling to the thumb, index, middle and half of the ring finger. Symptoms include tingling, pain or numbness in the hand and fingers.

"It's typically worse with reading a newspaper or book, talking on the phone or driving a car, and frequently it wakes people up in the middle of the night with tingling or pain in the hand," says Benn Smith, M.D., co-author of the study and neurologist at Mayo Clinic in Scottsdale, Arizona.

"Very often, people obtain temporary relief by shaking the hand or rubbing it, causing the numbness and tingling to go away."

There are a variety of factors that contribute to Carpal Tunnel Syndrome (CTS). "The major risk factors for developing carpal tunnel syndrome are being female and middle-aged," says J. Clarke Stevens, M.D., a neurologist at Mayo Clinic in Rochester, Minnesota. "There are many other causes of carpal tunnel syndrome, such as wrist trauma, diabetes, rheumatoid arthritis and pregnancy."

Repetitive motions in industries outside the office also have been linked to CTS, Dr. Stevens says. "There have been a number of studies of factory workers and people in packing plants that suggest that type of repetitive motion does seem to be associated with carpal tunnel syndrome."

The biggest problem with carpal tunnel syndrome is that it is highly over-diagnosed.

Doctors unfamiliar with trigger point and referred pain theory often overlook the true causes of problems in the areas associated with carpal tunnel and leap to erroneous conclusions.

The most common reasons for misdiagnosis of CTS are weakness in the annular ligament of the elbow, or referred pain from cervical vertebrae to the thumb, index and middle fingers.

A problematic annular ligament when pressed may be a trigger point to the carpal tunnel distribution in the hand.

Once the annular ligament is injected with Prolotherapy or trigger point therapy, it is often deactivated and the symptoms of carpal tunnel syndrome disappear.

Traditional methods of treating carpal tunnel syndrome include wearing a splint at night or injections of cortisone to reduce swelling. If these measures are not successful, carpal tunnel release surgery, which sections the tough transverse carpal ligament and relieves pressure on the median nerve, may be performed. But as we have seen with arthroscopy for the knee, surgery should be the last treatment a patient should ever consider.

Countless patients have presented to my office with worse symptoms after they had the carpal tunnel surgery.

Prolotherapy to strengthen the annular ligament will often cure chronic elbow pain.

Under no circumstances should a patient consent to surgery for CTS until an evaluation is performed by a physician trained in the referral patterns of pain in ligaments.

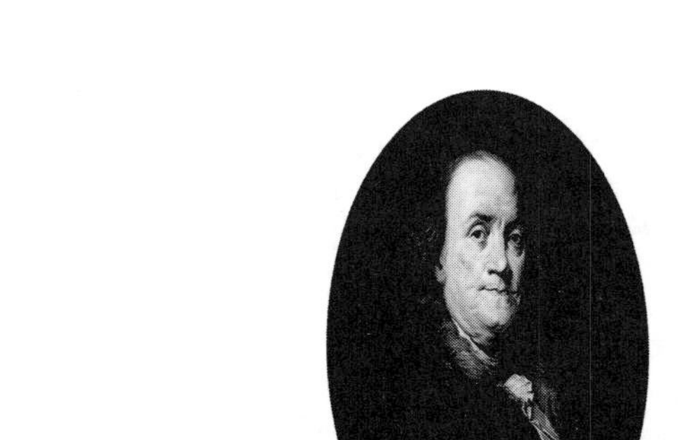

"Be sober and temperate,
and you will be healthy."
—Benjamin Franklin—

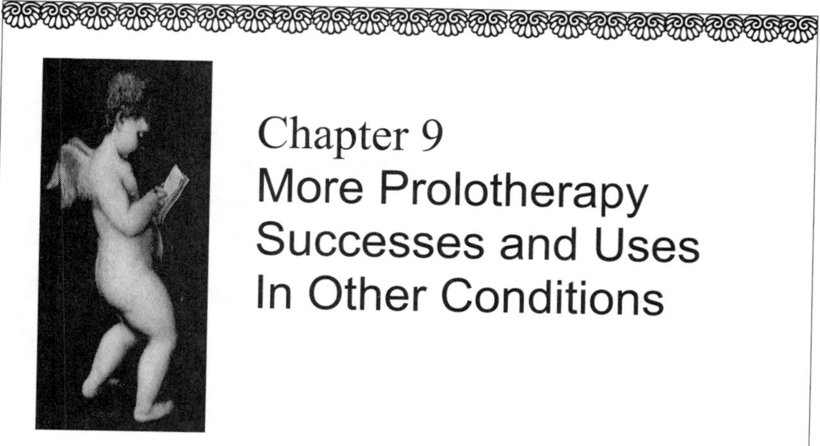

Chapter 9 More Prolotherapy Successes and Uses In Other Conditions

Throughout this book we have seen how Prolotherapy has helped many people with many different, painful conditions. Prolotherapy can also be helpful in notoriously difficult problems to treat: pain in the hip and pelvic area; pain from extreme contact sports like boxing, football, and wrestling, and pain caused by extreme gyration, like that of trapeze artists. Later in this chapter we will also discuss other conditions such as head, neck and jaw pain.

Lamon Brewster, A Champion Has Numerous Pains

Just saying that Lamon is a boxer should be all the convincing anyone would need that he was an excellent candidate for Prolotherapy. Boxing is a violent sport that puts tremendous stress on the body. This was attested to by Lamon's first visit to Joint Rehabilitation in 2001.

Lamon told me that his knee caps felt loose and that his knees had been hurting him for over two years. He also had right shoulder pain and right pectoralis tenderness and lower back pain.

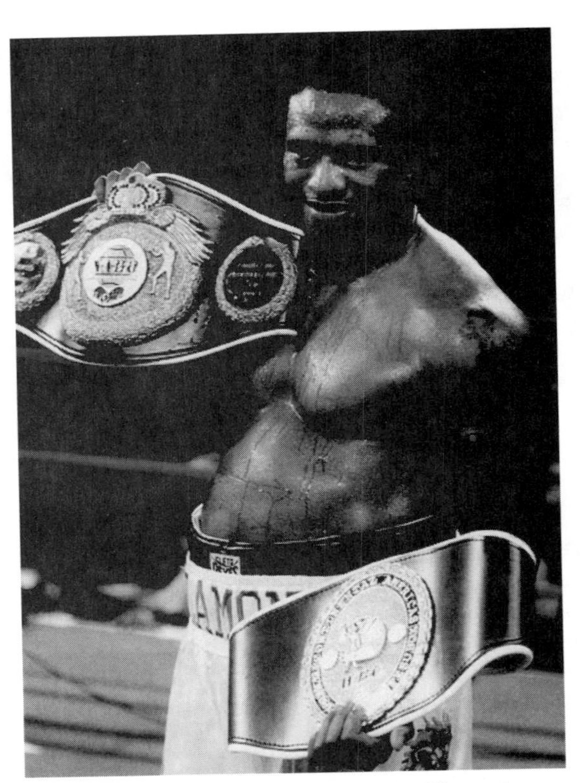

Lamon Brewster, Heavyweight Champion

We put Prolotherapy right to work on him, first on the right pectoralis muscle on the lateral side that Lamon injured while sparring. "I don't think that I was warmed up quite as well as I should have," says Lamon, "(when I threw a punch) I just felt everything rip in my shoulder on the right side." We also injected Lamon's knees and back: The results?

"I was able to jab and get back in the ring within three weeks whereas, that is the type of injury that I think that would have put aside my career for at least three months. That was one of

the best recoveries I ever had. But it was just not my shoulder, everything, like my knees, **is 100% better**. I mean, it really got better, you know, my back as well."

Even when winning, you can get hurt in boxing. Lamon suffered a wrist injury when hitting an opponent who was on the way down. "My left hand, the metacarpals, I had a guy that I hit his forehead with an upper cut as he was falling." Lamon's wrist was injected twice.

"You know me being an athlete, I associate with a ton of athletes and I always tell them about Prolotherapy. This is something that I wish more people knew about before they would go to a doctor, because the first thing the doctor wants to do is cut on you or he wants to give you some type of medicine. I can't afford to sit around for six months waiting for something to heal. I need that right now, and the Prolotherapy is the 'right now' cure for me."

Lamon is also an actor, you may have seen Lamon in the Ben Affleck movie "Daredevil," and on TV in "Martin" and "Ally McBeal."

Mr. Universe's Blown-Out Hip, Joe DeAngelis

"While preparing for a bodybuilding competition still six weeks away, I was in the middle of an intense leg workout. Squats were part of the routine that day, topping out with a descending set from 700 pounds.

I was on my second 'rep' with 700 pounds, it was at the bottom of the movement when I felt my hip literally explode. I stayed stuck at the bottom, and now realize that I went into shock almost immediately. I fell, but eventually pulled myself to my feet. My leg went numb, and I knew something serious had happened.

In the days that followed, my leg turned black and blue. I never considered backing out of the show, and did my best to train around the injury. Sitting and standing were unbearable. In the few days following the injury, my wife had to help me dress. Getting in and out of the car became a dreaded experience.

After the competition, the injury stayed aggravated. Even after the most feeble leg workouts I would be limping for hours. I developed a baseball sized rock-hard lump on the side of my thigh. After about six months of this pain, I was introduced to Dr. Darrow at the ***Joint Rehabilitation and Sports Medical Center, Inc***.

Dr. Darrow told me the trigger point effect of his injections might relieve the pain, but there was nothing he could do to reduce the lump on my hip. Additionally, the possible Prolotherapy effect might even grow some new collagen and assist the healing.

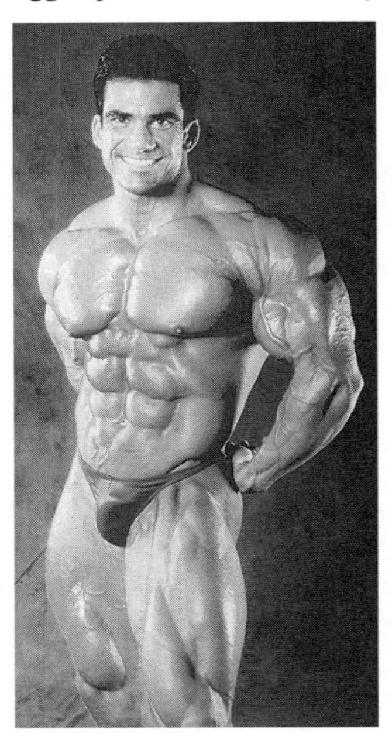

Joe DeAngelis

I didn't care if it was trigger points or Prolotherapy because the results were miraculous.

After six months of pain and the inability to squat 225, I performed repetitions with 500 pounds!

This was after only four treatments. Not only that, but that big rock on my thigh disappeared. Now I'm back to (working out with) 700 pounds.

While I never admit even to myself how bad the situation may have been, there was always the feeling that those heavy days of squatting and dead-lifting were over for good. Prolotherapy literally gave me a new lease on my training life."

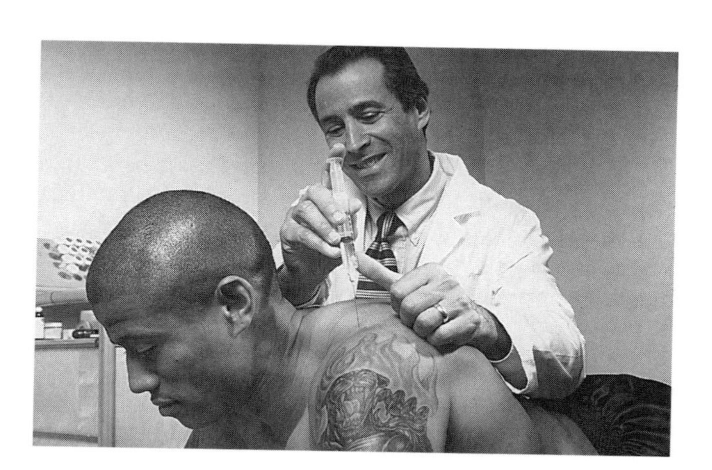

Dr. Darrow gives Prolotherapy to the NFL's Johnnie Morton, Jr.

A Football Player and Pelvic Pain

Johnnie Morton Jr., is a professional football player. A wide receiver for the Detroit Lions and Kansas City Chiefs. Originally he was pessimistic about trying Prolotherapy. He just happened to be in my office escorting a friend who was undergoing treatment. Johnnie figured he had tried every kind of therapy in the book for his chronic pain.

He is a top athlete on a professional football team in the NFL. He figured the team's trainers and doctors had every available resource at their disposal to treat his pain and injuries, right?

"Dr. Darrow's needle feels like an angel dancing on my skin. His treatment gave me my first pain free season in ten years."

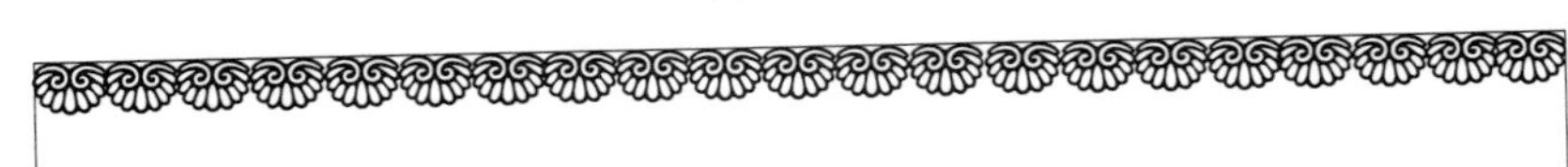

Nothing had worked before. Sure he had some temporary relief, but he thought living with pain was an inevitable price you paid in professional sports. He was understandably skeptical at trying another therapy.

Thankfully, my power of persuasion must have been on that day. After talking to Johnnie he agreed to try Prolotherapy. Johnnie suffered from both a painful sprain where the gluteus muscle attaches to the pelvis and a badly sprained thumb joint from getting clipped during games.

After only two Prolotherapy sessions on each trigger point, Johnnie played his first pain-free season in ten years.

He was so pleased with the results that he now comes to me first with whatever ails him, and is referring other athletes to me for care.

It is important to understand that the actual initial relief Johnnie obtained was from the trigger point effect of the injections not the proliferation of collagen (see the next chapter on trigger points). Prolotherapy implies proliferation of collagen, a process that takes six-to-eight weeks to heal. Most of the time when a patient receives Prolotherapy he or she is benefiting from the trigger point injection effect, which can often be immediate.

Turf Toe

One of Johnnie's referrals was his then teammate David Sloan. David was the starting tight end for the Detroit Lions. In addition to David's skill on the field, he was voted one of *Muscle & Fitness NFL's Best Physiques* in October of 1999. When David came to me in the Spring of 2001, he suffered from metarsalgia, commonly known as "turf toe."

Metarsalgia is a painful condition resulting from training on the turf. While running, the foot gets repeatedly caught on the turf and jams the structures in the big toe.

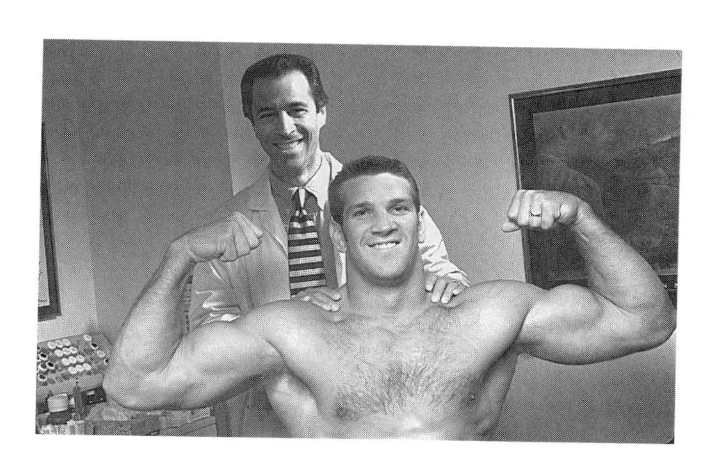

Dr. Darrow with footballer David Sloan

Jack Armstrong, "The Wildman's" Knees, Shoulder, and Hands

"Wildman" Jack Armstrong ranks among professional wrestling's greatest. In a career that spanned 29 years, Jack appeared in over 4,500 matches, his last coming in 1994.

Jack first came to our offices in late 2003 with complaints that would be expected of a retired wrestler.

"My knees were terrible (bone-on-bone arthritis and calcification). I wasn't able to sleep, so I went to an orthopedic physician and got some temporary relief from Hyalgan injections, but after 10 weeks the pain came back."

To help add longevity to his wrestling career, Jack ran marathons.

"I did 11 marathons. Every time you train for a marathon you are actually running 300 miles (practicing for it.)

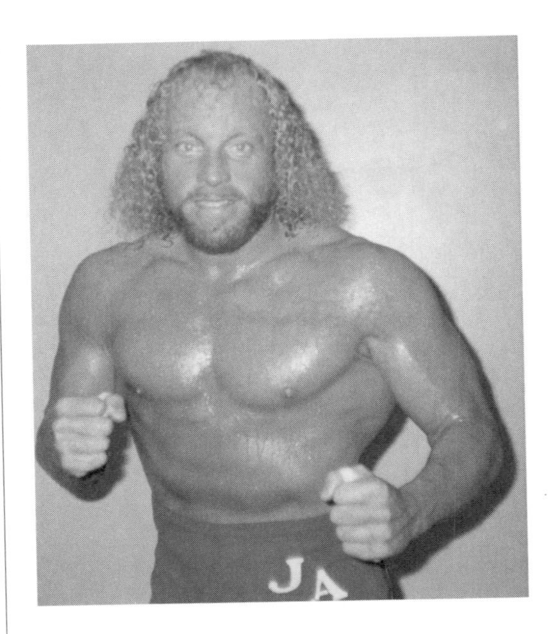

The "Wildman"

So, I wore my joints away (running) and smashed my joints wrestling.

"(Add to this a recent accident), I fell off a horse. My right shoulder (was terrible), I couldn't put on a shirt or go to sleep. My right hand (was terrible), I wasn't even able to lift an orange juice without shooting pain. Same with the equipment in the gym, which only weighs seven or eight pounds. I couldn't hold it."

It didn't take long for Jack to see some startling results and an alleviation of his pain.

"Prolotherapy works like a miracle! If you have a problem, take advantage (of this) before going to surgery. Since I have been getting Prolotherapy with Dr. Darrow I have been checking out people who had knee surgeries, back surgeries, etc. I say to them, 'How do you feel? You had L4-5 done, how do you feel?' They would say, 'Terrible.' I would ask, 'How do you feel when it

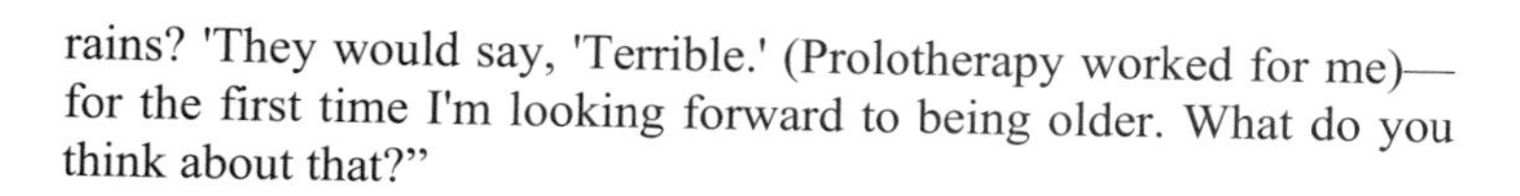

rains? 'They would say, 'Terrible.' (Prolotherapy worked for me)—for the first time I'm looking forward to being older. What do you think about that?"

A Letter From The Trapeze

October 16, 2003
Marc Darrow, MD, JD
Joint Rehabilitation and Sports Medical Center

Dear Marc,

I am writing on behalf of my team (The Flying Farfans) to express our gratitude and thank you and your staff for providing us over the years with Prolotherapy.

Our profession takes us all over the world and our work is quite demanding physically. Due to the extreme stress load our bodies endure as aerial acrobats, aches and pains is just part of our livelihood.

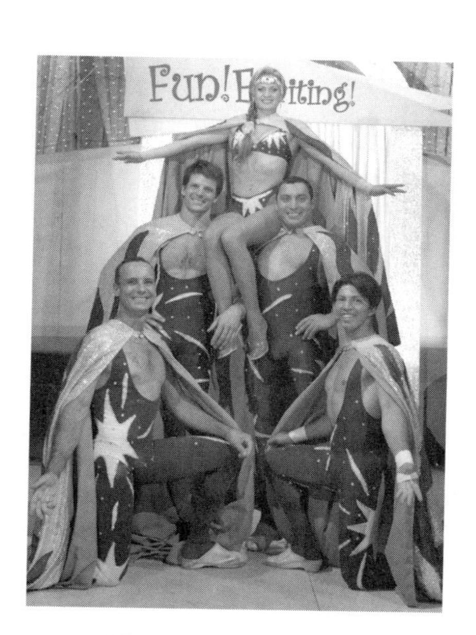

That's Gino on the left.

I have been using Prolotherapy for many years now and have referred my team as well since 1999. At first, none of my teammates had ever heard of Prolotherapy and everyone was excited since chiropractic care, massage and other forms of body treatment had never quite worked for them.

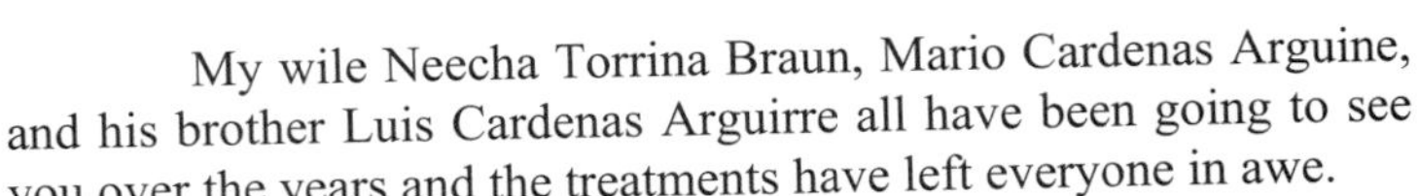

My wile Neecha Torrina Braun, Mario Cardenas Arguine, and his brother Luis Cardenas Arguirre all have been going to see you over the years and the treatments have left everyone in awe.

We are all so grateful to finally perform pain free again; there is nothing more enjoyable than flying thru the air with ease, and not having to force a smile on our faces because the severe pain we endured.

Doctor Darrow, you have made our lives so much easier and your treatments have truly worked wonders for all of us. There are no words to express the difference it makes in one's life to be able to go through the day without feeling under the weather because of pain.

We will continue using Prolotherapy for years to come because it is simply the best cure for us, the daring young men on the flying trapeze.

Truly yours,
Gino Farfan

Headaches & Neck Pain

Although the common headache usually responds quite well to aspirin or other over-the-counter medications, those who have experienced the torment of migraines or cluster headaches are often frustrated by the lack of any effective cure. Drugs developed specifically for such headaches may be effective, but the relief they provide is temporary. Until the root of the problem is unearthed and corrected, the headaches will persist, and prolonged drug therapy to relieve them will be necessary, along with the possibility of addiction.

In rare cases, the problem is traced to cysts or brain tumors, but more often it is related to muscular or ligamentary tension. Most people know the phrase "tension headache" but not many—doctors included—are aware that neck tendons and ligaments refer pain directly to the head. In cases where no cyst or tumor is found but headaches persist, Prolotherapy may be in order.

A physician skilled in diagnosing trigger points and recognizing referred pain signals should be consulted in such cases.

In one famous case, Prolotherapist Gustav Hemwall, M.D., treated NBA basketball star Kendall Gill for headache pain that had persisted for 16 years. Pain pills and injections of painkillers provided transitory relief, but the headaches always returned "with a vengeance" in the words of the long-suffering athlete.

After a single treatment with Prolotherapy, Gill was headache-free for two years!

BARRÉ-LIEOU SYNDROME

Barré-Lieou Syndrome is characterized by a grab bag of diverse symptoms, all of which are rooted in the sympathetic nervous system, specifically the cluster of nerves located in the posterior cervical area at the back of the neck. It is caused when the sympathetic nerves are pinched by loose, weakly supported vertebrae. These nerves are part of the autonomic nervous system that regulates the body's functions, a myriad of activities ranging from such critical functions as your heartbeat and breathing to countless minor ones.

A list of problems that may be due to Barré-Lieou Syndrome:

Headache	**Sinusitis**	**Allergies**
Dizziness	**Neck Pain**	**Chest Pain**
Face Pain	**Eye Pain**	**Blurred Vision**
Ear Pain	**Tinnitus**	**Hoarseness**
Laryngitis	**Fatigue**	**Vertigo**

If you have any of those symptoms, combined with neck pain, you may be a candidate for Prolotherapy.

TEMPOROMANDIBULAR JOINT SYNDROME (TMJ)

The temporomandibular joint is where the jaw meets the cranium. The condition known as temporomandibular joint syndrome develops from a combination of interrelated factors, usually starting with poor head posture that contributes to the stretching and weakening of the cervical ligaments and lateral TMJ ligaments. As a result, the lower jaw slips forward, aggravating the situation further by putting additional stress on the ligaments and the joints.

One characteristic of TMJ is the loud popping or clicking of ligaments or bones rubbing together in the loosened joint, accompanied by pain and stiffness as the muscles tighten, trying to compensate for the instigating laxity.

Conventional treatments include TMJ arthroscopy and various types of surgery, TMJ implants, injections of botulinum toxin, and cauterization. All of these are invasive and somewhat risky, and treat the immediate problem while largely ignoring future consequences.

Prolotherapy is a highly effective treatment for TMJ Syndrome, particularly when the related neck ligaments are treated along with the TMJ ligaments.

By strengthening these two sets of ligaments, Prolotherapy can eliminate not only the existing TMJ (and any neck-related) problems, but also helps to circumvent recurrences as well.

In Summary

In summary, if you suffer from chronic pain and/or any connective tissue trauma or injury, before you succumb to any last resort treatments such as surgery, cortisone injections or other so called conventional therapies, you owe it to yourself to find a Prolotherapist and discuss your options. After all, as I have said over and over again, it is safe, effective and relatively inexpensive.

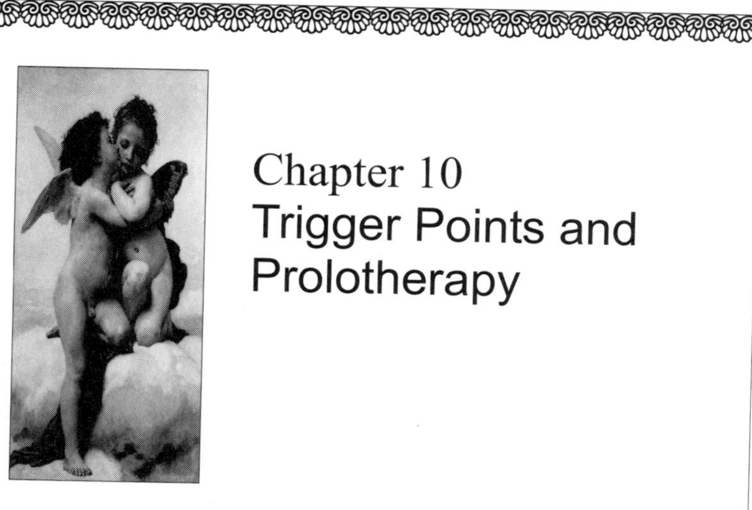

Chapter 10
Trigger Points and Prolotherapy

A normal healthy body contains an intricate framework of bones and cartilage supported in perfect harmony by a network of semi-elastic tissues, mainly tendons and ligaments. Dysfunction in these tissues can cause a wide variety of problems.

When the tendons or ligaments, which anchor the structure, are weakened or damaged, the stress and friction created by the misalignment of joints results in chronic pain, and over the years, arthritis in many cases. Similar stresses can be caused by the action of dysfunctional muscles, tendons, or ligaments containing problem areas known as "trigger points" or "tender points"—hyperirritable, painful soft tissue areas.

Direct Muscle Pain and Referred Pain

Injury or disease can cause pain in muscles. The spot of muscle tissue injury causing pain is called the active trigger point. Now just because the active trigger point causes the pain does not mean that the spot is painful itself. When the pain causing spot is painful it is called a primary trigger point. However pain can also manifest in distant areas away from the active trigger point. Such pain is called referred pain.

Secondary Trigger Point

Secondary trigger points are painful spots in a muscle or fascia (the thin layer that helps separate one muscle from another) that became painful because the muscle it's in has a working relationship with the muscle that contained the primary trigger point.

Satellite Trigger Point

A satellite trigger point is simply one that receives pain because it is located in a zone of reference linked directly to the active trigger point, an area known as the essential pain zone. There are also areas known as spill-over pain zones that receive pain signals that spill out beyond the normal boundaries of the essential pain zone where it originates.

Besides the pain caused by active trigger points, there are symptoms other than pain that are caused by latent trigger points. Some common latent symptoms include weakness, stiffness or restriction of movement. Both active and latent trigger points cause dysfunction—but only active ones cause pain.

Myofasciitis *is a general term used to describe pain or other dysfunctions in the network of muscles, tendons, and ligaments and other soft connective tissue that holds our bodies together.*

Myofascial pain may start abruptly or gradually. Abrupt onset is usually the result of trauma to the muscle, such as a sudden overload or over-extension, while a gradual onset is due to chronic overload, virus, or other disease, or psychogenic stress.

Through an understanding of the various symptoms of pain, such as whether it occurs at rest or during activity, what muscles it is related to, whether it is primary or referred, and countless other factors, the doctor can isolate the problem and treat it with a technique known as trigger point therapy.

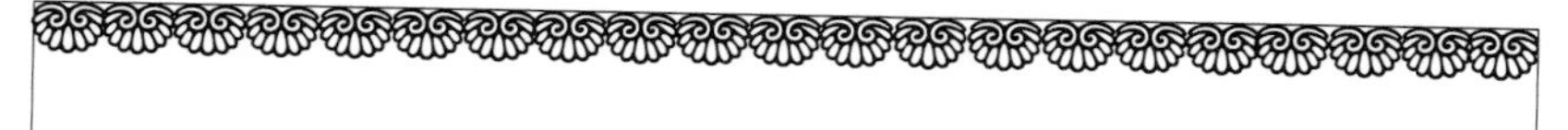

A Brief History of Trigger Point Therapy

Trigger point therapy is a fairly modern science which developed as a result of decades of observation and studies into the nature of pain by researchers around the world. Various techniques of therapy blossomed with each new revelation, evolving from deep massage to the needle therapies (i.e., acupuncture, trigger point, or Prolotherapy) used today.

The German physician Froriep took the first recorded steps in the trigger point arena in 1843. He coined the phrase "muskel-schwiele" (muscle callouses) to identify the hard cords found in muscle tissue in cases of rheumatic pain.

Other physicians adopted his ideas and continued studying the problem of muscle pain based on his assumption. But by the end of the century, one of his countrymen debunked the theory on the grounds that no real "callouses" of deposited material were found in these tender muscles.

Although German physicians held the lead for many years to come, Swedish and British researchers conducted their own studies and offered their own contributions, with the same mixed results.

American researchers in the 1930's were among the first to describe instances of referred pain, and a major breakthrough was achieved in 1939 when British researchers Kellgren and Lewis proved that the previously held, but not widely accepted notion of referred pain, was indeed rooted in fact. But even their observations were limited by the then rudimentary understanding of the complexities of the spine and nervous system.

Other brilliant researchers came forth with major findings shortly thereafter. Polish physician Gutstein, writing first in German, and later in English (as Gutstein-Good), after relocating to Great Britain, advanced the concept of trigger points, which he called "myalgic spots," as well as the importance of analyzing the patient's pain reaction, later called the "jump sign." Contributing over a dozen papers between 1938 and 1957, his observations on trigger points were highly astute, and steered his colleagues in the proper direction.

OCCIPITO–CERVICAL DISABILITY

LIGAMENT AND TENDON RELAXATION

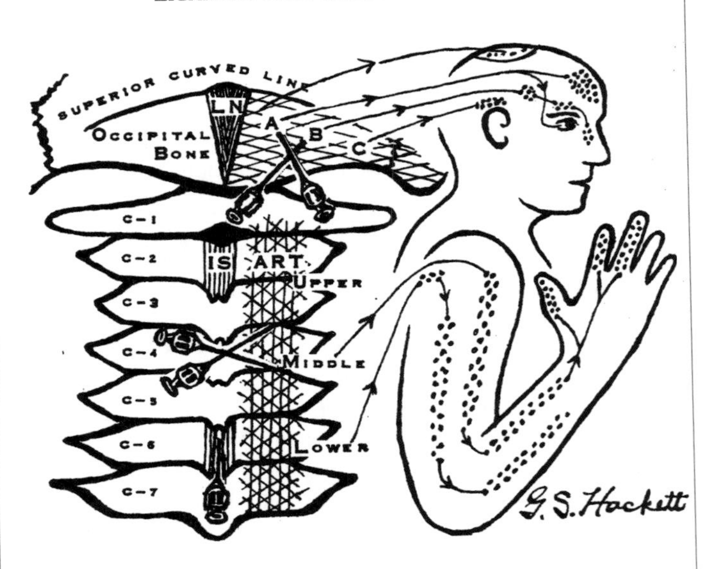

TRIGGER POINTS — REFERRED PAIN AREAS

POSITION OF NEEDLES FOR DIAGNOSIS AND TREATMENT

OCCIPITAL TENDONS

REFERRED PAIN, HEADACHE, DIZZINESS

A – FOREHEAD, EYE

B – TEMPLE, EYEBROW, NOSE

C – ABOVE EAR

CERVICAL LIGAMENTS

IS – INTERSPINUS LIGAMENTS

ART – ARTICULAR LIGAMENTS

REFERRED PAIN

UPPER – NECK

MIDDLE – ARM, FOREARM, THUMB,
1 AND 2 FINGERS

LOWER – ACROMIUM PROCESS, ARM,
FOREARM

FIG. 25

Hans Kraus introduced a great advancement in the treatment of muscle pain in 1937 when he pioneered the use of vapocoolant spray to treat muscle pain and relieve trigger points. In 1970, Kraus published a book on the beneficial effects of exercise on patients with back pain.

Janet G. Travell, M.D., reached prominence as the personal physician to Presidents John F. Kennedy and Lyndon Baines Johnson. David Simons, M.D., was a U.S. Air Force flight surgeon conducting experiments in the nascent field of Aerospace Medical Research when he and Travell met at the School of Aerospace Medicine.

Together they produced one of the most comprehensive reference manuals in the history of pain medicine, "Myofascial Pain and Dysfunction: The Trigger Point Manual," an exhaustive presentation covering every practical aspect of trigger point therapy. It included descriptions of techniques and ingredients to maps of all the known trigger point reference patterns.

Diagnostic procedures include testing for taut bands of muscle fiber, twitch response, and applied pressure to check for referred pain triggers. There is evidence to suggest that trigger points are caused by impaired circulation and/or an increased metabolic demand.

Skeletal muscle tissue accounts for about 40% of our body weight, and includes nearly 700 individual muscles. When active trigger points are present, passive or active stretching of the muscle produces pain. This pain can occur with the slightest activity or even at rest. Biofeedback has proven that muscles are in a state of contraction and activity even when we believe we are at rest.

When myofascial pain is related to a single muscle trauma, or exhibits a stable pattern over any length of time, it is usually easy to diagnose and treat.

In cases where pain appears in multiple muscles, spreads to other areas, or there is evidence of increasing fibrosis or other

contributing factors, pain can be very difficult to diagnose and treat.

Once the proper diagnosis is ascertained, however, various treatments are available to deal with the problem effectively.

Knowledge of the referred pain pattern characteristic of each muscle is often the most important single source of information used in diagnosing pain.

The patient's examination begins with observation of their posture, movements, body structure and symmetry. It progresses with specialized screening movements to isolate the problem areas and identify trigger points.

However, tendons, ligaments and joint capsules may also refer pain to areas distant from the actual trigger point. Tender points, which are points that are sore with pressure or palpation of the doctor's hand, may also be treated with trigger point injections or Prolotherapy. Unlike the dry needle of acupuncture, the trigger point or Prolotherapy needles deliver fluid to the target area to be treated. By puncturing the tissue, trauma to the area is caused, resulting in a rush of white blood cells to the area that provokes an anti-inflammatory reaction and stimulates the healing process. Frequently, in trigger point therapy the physician will use a local anesthetic solution such as lidocaine to relieve the pain as well.

The deep tissue injection of the trigger point attacks the problem directly, causing physical changes and subsequent, histological composition of the tissue provoked by the needle.

Prolotherapy takes trigger point theory a step further, by adding an irritant solution, like dextrose or phenol to the injection process.

This irritant solution helps speed up the proliferation of new collagen tissue.

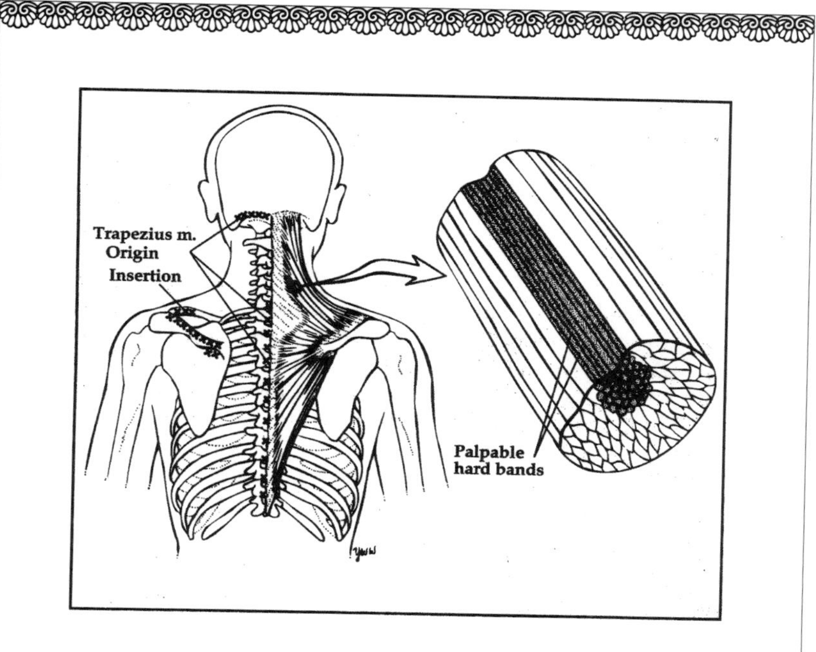

It is highly effective for rejuvenation of joints, muscles, tendons and ligaments. Acupuncture, trigger point therapy, and Prolotherapy are basically variations of the same therapeutic process, all originating from ancient medical arts, best known in China and Greece.

Yet despite the overwhelming evidence of its effectiveness, Prolotherapy has yet to achieve full acceptance by the medical community.

Perhaps it is because, as Dr. William Faber, Director of the Milwaukee Pain Clinic and a leading authority in the field of Prolotherapy, points out, "...the substances used in Prolotherapy are not patented and therefore would not provide the huge profits that pharmaceutical therapies receive."

Nevertheless, the big companies have nothing patented in the field of trigger point therapy or acupuncture, both of which are accepted today.

Could it be that there is a resistance to Prolotherapy because it would substantially reduce the number of surgeries?

If this is the case, it is a sad comment on our dollar driven medical system. Without all of the unnecessary surgeries, would hospitals go out of business?

Prolotherapy also requires specialized training, sometimes with long needles, and only a few hundred physicians have made the commitment to master the procedure. But based on the public demand, this is about to change.

The Natural Healing Cascade

In order to fully appreciate how Prolotherapy works, it is essential to understand the natural healing process that it mimics, known in the world of medicine as "the natural healing cascade."

This process is complex, but has been extensively studied by the medical community and is readily understood.

When an injury occurs to a muscle, joint, tendon or ligament, or loss of fluid in the body through aging or illness causes a weakening of these tissues, it becomes inflamed, or irritated.

This irritation provokes a defensive immune response and sequestering of fibroblasts into the damaged area. These cells produce the miraculous healing compound collagen.

Absorbed into and around the damaged tissue, the collagen builds up and fortifies these structures. It then shrinks and stabilizes. After proliferative therapy, a ligament can become 50% thicker and 200-400% stronger.

It is interesting to consider that inflammation is the inciting factor that actually stimulates the entire healing process.

In his massive and scholarly tome, ***"Prolo Your Sports Injury Away,"*** Dr. Ross Hauser suggests a very intriguing theory about inflammation and sports injuries.

Sports injuries are commonly "treated" with an injection of steroids—which are administered specifically for their anti-inflammatory effect. Hauser wonders if recurring sports injuries aren't in fact caused by this routine use of steroid injections—which by their very nature would interfere with the body's ability to produce fibroblasts and therefore to produce the collagen it sorely needs to repair and strengthen its damaged tissue.

If this indeed proves to be true, then the decision to choose Prolotherapy over corticosteroid injections could mean the difference between a record-breaking career and or a career-breaking decision.

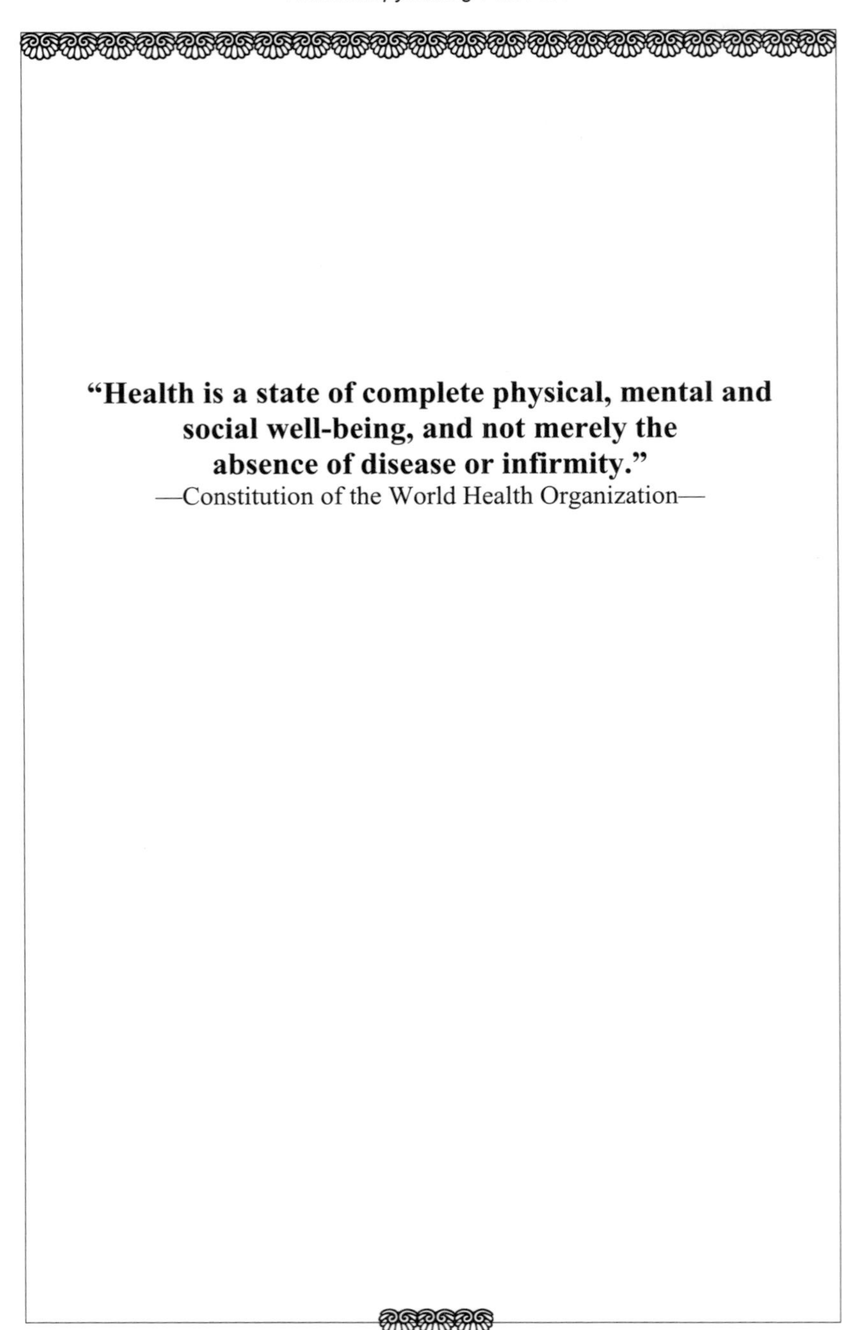

"Health is a state of complete physical, mental and social well-being, and not merely the absence of disease or infirmity."

—Constitution of the World Health Organization—

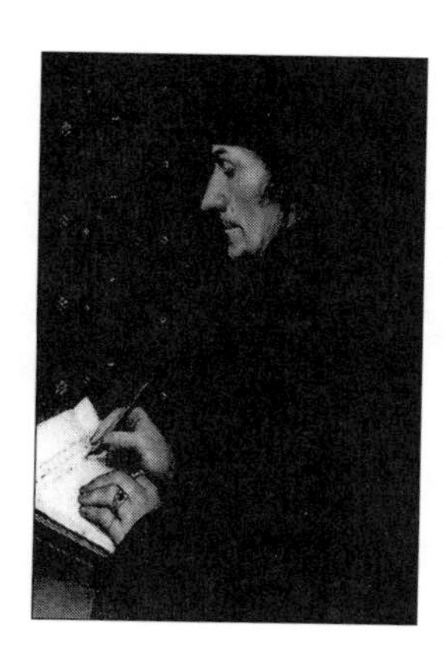

Chapter 11
And Even More Success Stories

Marc Darrow, M.D.,
Joint Rehabilitation & Sports Medical Center
Los Angeles, CA 90025

Dear Dr. Darrow:

Prolo works! After injuring my shoulder (hyperextension/overuse syndrome) near the tail end of the Long Drive competitive season, I was beginning to wonder if it would ever get back to normal. Progress was inching along at a snail's pace when I was utilizing massage, heat, icing, manipulation, and various rehabilitative exercises.

After only one injection, my shoulder was probably 80% recovered after three days. I could do most of the upper body exercises I used to do prior to the injury, and was pain free with my golf swing. I found that very impressive.

After receiving treatment on both my right shoulder, which was the one originally injured, and the left one, which I wanted healed as well, the long drive season started again. Prior to my injury, my best drive was 385 yards. After my injury, but before treatment, I was incapable of hitting over 300 yards. In my first

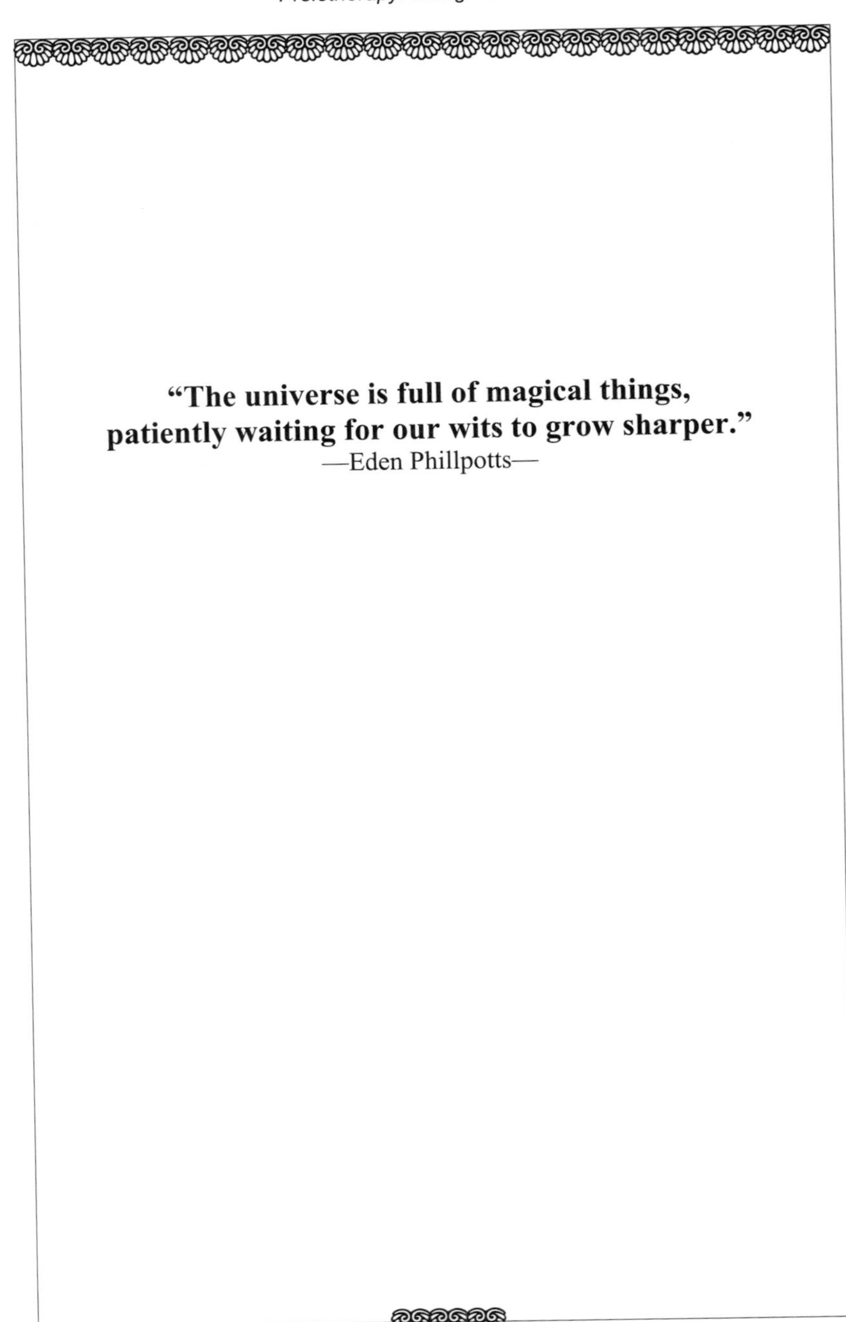

"The universe is full of magical things, patiently waiting for our wits to grow sharper."
—Eden Phillpotts—

event after treatment, hitting a standard length club to ease into the competition again, I hit a 320 yard drive. I have already qualified for the Southern California District and I feel absolutely no pain in either shoulder. It's pretty amazing."

My gratitude to you,

Name Omitted

Although there may have been an additional proliferative effect, the quick healing seemed to be from the trigger point effect of the injections.

Marc Darrow, M.D., J.D.
Joint Rehabilitation and Sports Medical Center
Los Angeles, CA 90025

To Dr. Darrow:

I would like to convey the following results of our Prolo therapy experience. I first saw you in January of this year for a chronic and very painful hip problem. At first I was very leery and scared about doing the injections. In the end the pain and discomfort got to me and I agreed to the injections. We had two sessions. After the first, the pain was signifi-cantly diminished. After the second session to date, the pain has not recurred. My daily life has so improved I can now walk for hours with no problems, and have gone back to aerobics three times a week. I would like to thank you and acknowledge your "gift."

Sincerely,
Name Omitted

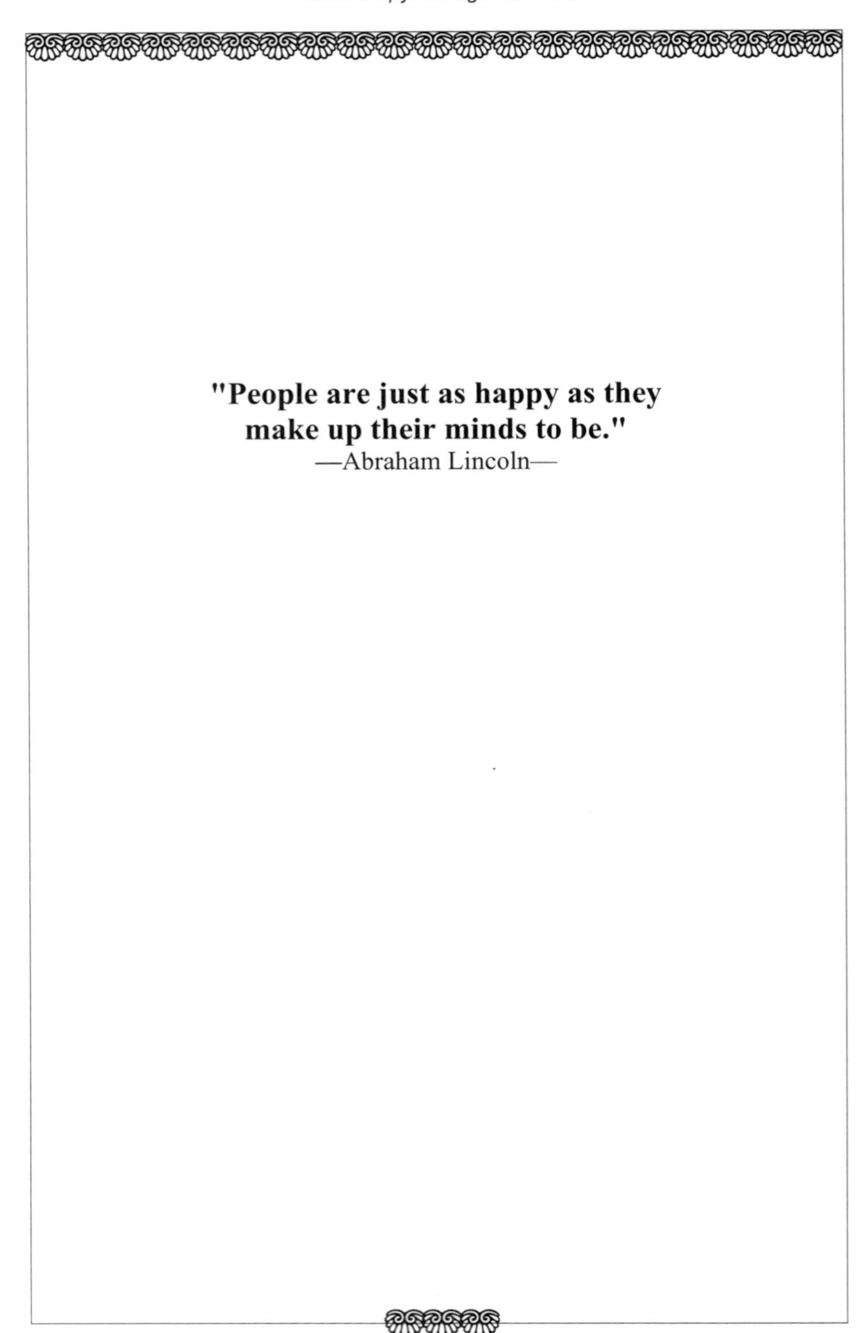

"People are just as happy as they make up their minds to be."
—Abraham Lincoln—

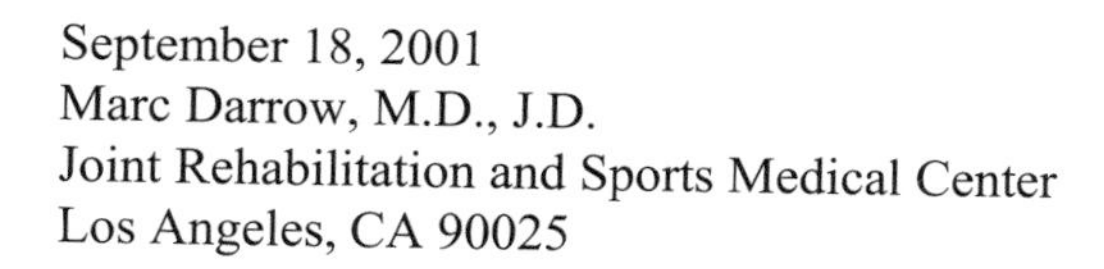
September 18, 2001
Marc Darrow, M.D., J.D.
Joint Rehabilitation and Sports Medical Center
Los Angeles, CA 90025

Dear Dr. Darrow:

I am so glad to have met you earlier this year. Last year I injured my right shoulder while playing tennis. For months I tried to let it heal by itself, but to no avail. I had pain doing simple tasks such as combing my hair or reaching for my wallet. I finally relented and saw an orthopedist who had it x-rayed. He concluded I had arthritis and there was nothing he could do. I was pretty upset because at age 43 I felt I had many years left to play tennis. That's when I met you. You said you could fix it with a weekly series of Prolotherapy injections. To make a long story short, you were correct. After seven treatments I was back on the court playing pain free.

However, as you know, that terrific state of affairs didn't last long. Two weeks later I tore two ligaments in my right ankle stepping on a tennis ball while going for a cross-court backhand shot. It blew up like a balloon. After I got an MRI the orthopedist said I would probably need surgery. I told him about you and that I wanted to see what you thought first. We decided to give Prolotherapy a chance. That, combined with an ankle exercise board and heat treatments, and use surgery as a last resort. Well, once again, you worked your magic and two months later I'm back playing tennis with reckless abandon. I don't even need an ankle support. I couldn't be more pleased.

I think your book, The Collagen Revolution: Living Pain Free should be mandatory reading for anyone who suffers joint pain, no matter what their age. It sure opened my eyes. I plan on playing tennis for another 50 years or so. Thanks for your help Dr. Darrow.

Sincerely,
Bill Strong
Beverly Hills, California

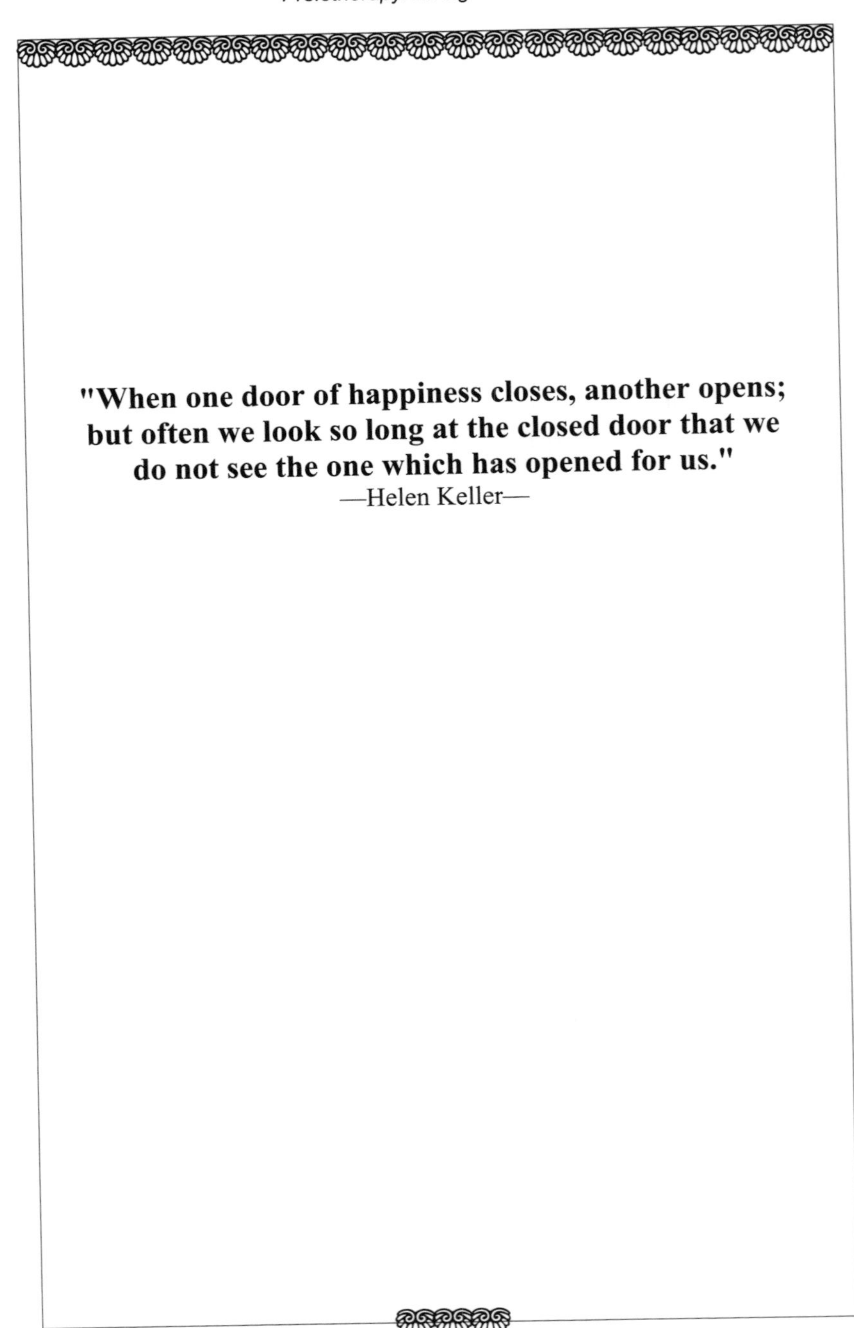

"When one door of happiness closes, another opens; but often we look so long at the closed door that we do not see the one which has opened for us."

—Helen Keller—

Marc Darrow, M.D.
Joint Rehabilitation
and Sports Medical Center
Los Angeles, CA 90025

Dr. Darrow:

I am so grateful to you, Dr. Bill, and Dr. Jason for helping me out of the chronic pain I had suffered with for so long. The injections were a godsend. My hip, lower back, ankle, and heel are 90% better. Thank you all for being so brave and innovative with your treatment.

Name Omitted

Marc Darrow, M.D., J.D.
Joint Rehabilitation
and Sports Medical Center
Los Angeles, CA 90025

Dr. Darrow:

Yippee, hooray, right on. Pain is gone. Prolo has me dancing again. My knee is healed.

Name Omitted

Marc Darrow, M.D.
Joint Rehabilitation and Sports Medical Center
Los Angeles, CA 90025

Dear Dr. Darrow:

Approximately six weeks ago I started Prolotherapy. I have had on and off back pain in the lower lumbar area for approximately 15 years. After a recent car accident the pain became very acute.

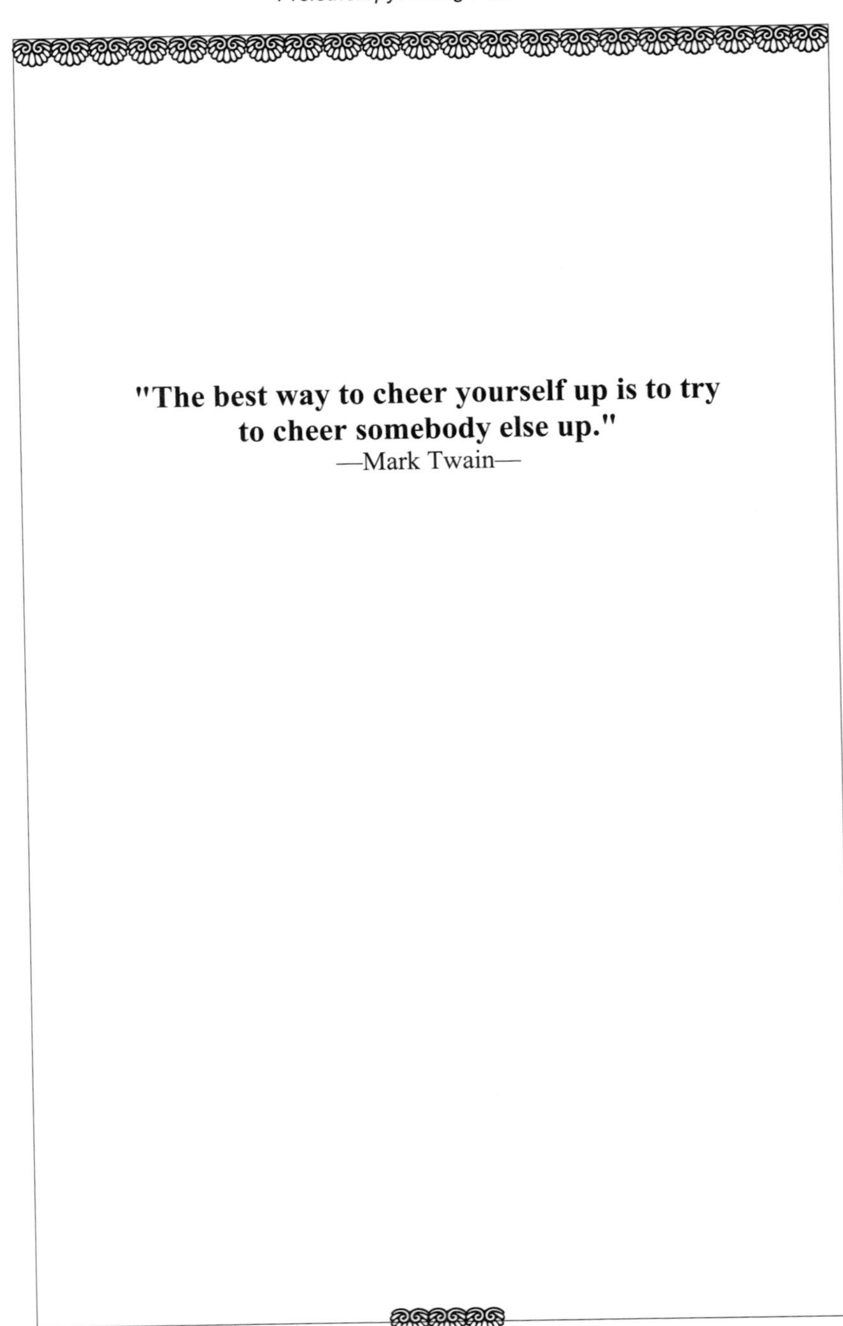

"The best way to cheer yourself up is to try to cheer somebody else up."
—Mark Twain—

After only three shots, the pain ceased altogether. But most amazingly, I started developing major shoulder pain that was very debilitating. After two shots with Prolo therapy the pain is totally gone. This pain was a deep ache that would bother me while driving a car. The results have been amazing.

Thank you,

Name Omitted

Marc Darrow, MD.
Joint Rehabilitation and
Sports Medical Center
Los Angeles, CA 90025

Dear Dr. Darrow:

On January 27,1999 I got into a car accident that injured my lower back. I tried everything from herbs to acupuncture. Everything seemed to do well, but being a dancer I am prone to re-injuring myself. After three months of misery, I finally decided to try Prolotherapy. It was a bit uncomfortable at first. It completely increased not only the strength, but gave me a sense of recovering that lies ahead. It was the strongest decision I have made for myself in my career and I don't think I could have continued dancing without it.

Sincerely,

Name Omitted

"Look at everything as though you were seeing it for the first time or last time. Then your time on earth will be filled with glory."

—A Tree Grows in Brooklyn—

Marc Darrow, M.D.
Joint Rehabilitation and
Sports Medical Center
Los Angeles, CA 90025

Dear Dr. Darrow:

I just wanted you to know how quickly my back problem is healing. When I came in to see you in incredible pain, bent over like the hunchback of Notre Dame, I didn't believe I would ever have a strong back after 25 years of intermittent spasms and lower back pain. Although its only couple of weeks since you injected me, 90% of the pain and weakness is gone. I can stand straight and feel more like I want to feel.

Very gratefully,

Name Omitted

Marc Darrow, MD.
Joint Rehabilitation and
Sports Medical Center
Los Angeles, CA 90025

Dr. Darrow:

I just wanted to let you know how pleased I am with my Prolo therapy. I spent almost the entire month of January in bed taking pain medication for my moderate to severe back pain. That month was very depressing for me. I finally stopped all pain meds except for Ibuprofen and tried to force myself to do things. Sometimes I felt well enough to go out, but often just the idea of driving the car kept me home.

On my first visit with you, you explained the whole process and told me I could begin after stopping the anti-inflammatory drugs for a few days. I went home and told my husband this simply sounded too good to be true.

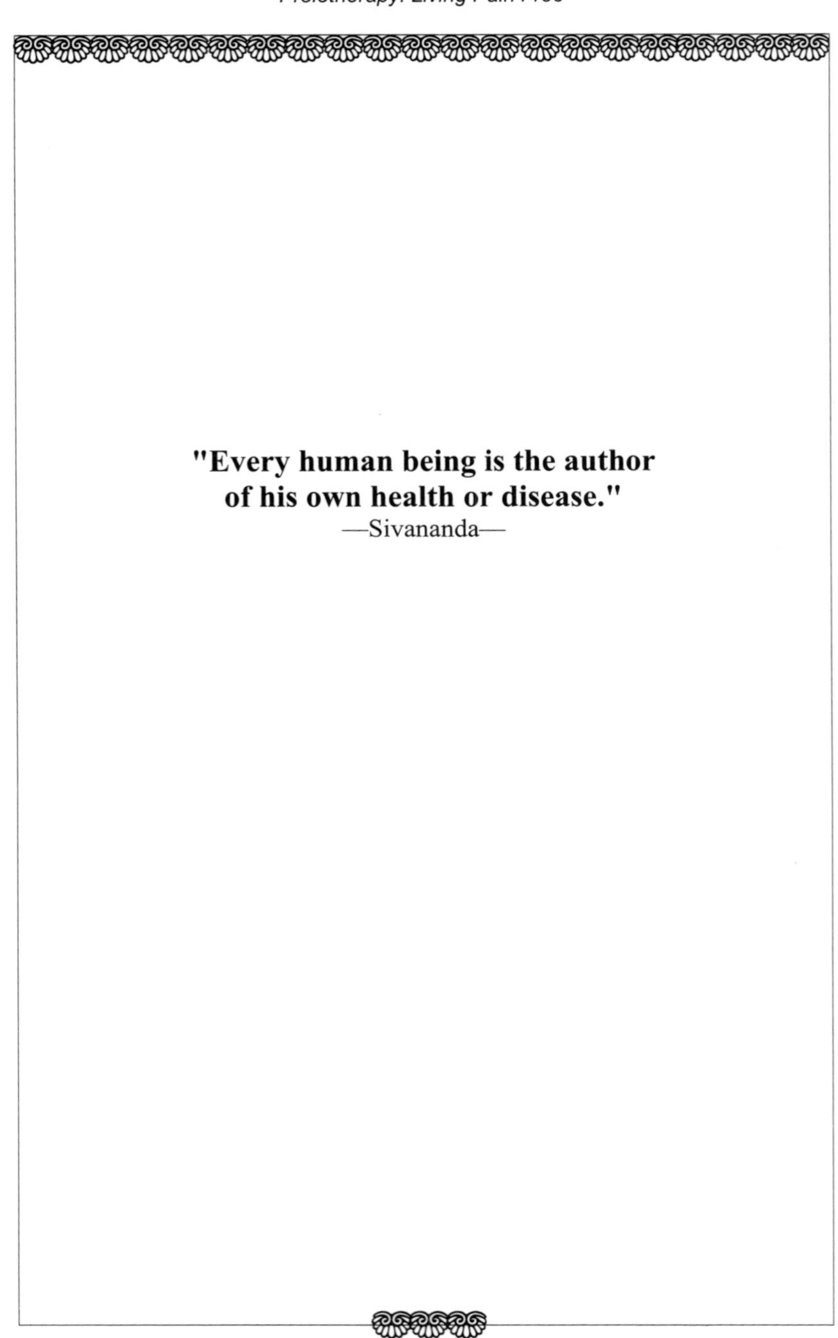

"Every human being is the author of his own health or disease."

—Sivananda—

I am a registered nurse with years of emergency room experience at UCLA Medical Center. I have suffered with back pain for 15 years. The idea that a series of dextrose injections could take away my pain and possibly keep it from reoccurring sounded ridiculous to me. To my surprise I was pain free after the first injection and have remained that way. I hope many patients will hear about the work you are doing and will be able to experience this "miracle." The whole approach of the clinic is great, the coordination with the other doctors, the exercise program, and the emphasis on wellness. Keep up the good work and thanks so much.

Name Omitted

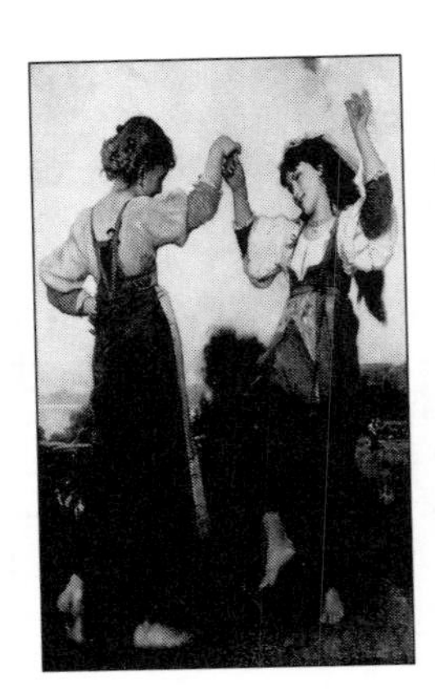

"The practice of forgiveness is our most important contribution to the healing of the world."
—Marianne Williamson—

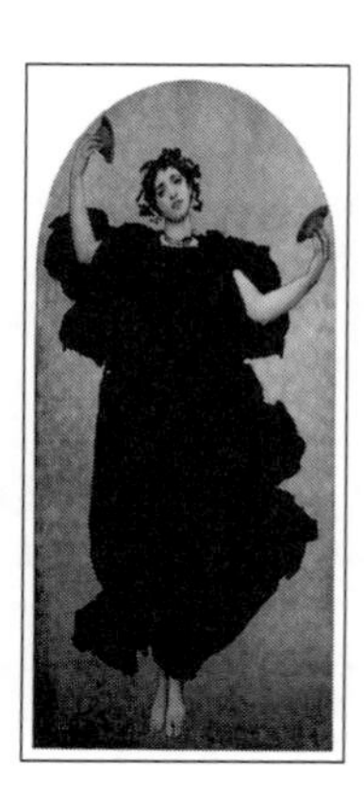

Chapter 12 The Doctor's Role in Healing

In every partnership, there must be trust. The only way trust can be formed is if a friendship is created. I truly care about what happens to my patients; both with their ailments and their life separate from that.

Once my patients become aware of this, they are able to place their trust in me and they are motivated to work with me, putting in their one hundred percent of the fifty percent of the work they committed to as we heal and head down the road to recovery.

I view only a small part of my job as the actual physical modalities. Yes, it is important to be technically correct as a physician. But, to me, that is just the beginning. Although patients are paying only for the procedural modalities, I make it my self-appointed responsibility to work on other levels. To do this I must truly listen and understand them. Not the easiest task in all cases, I must admit, and I certainly don't have it perfected.

You may be thinking, easier said than done, I agree. One of the first casualties in the battle between doctors and so-called

"managed care" insurers has been the doctor/patient relationship. The whole paradigm has shifted. Before managed care, the question was: ***What is best for the patient?*** After managed care the most pressing question for insurers is what is best for the bottom line? This has lead to an unhealthy state of affairs and leaves both doctors and patients frustrated.

Doctors are frustrated that they have to get approval for treatment from accountants who have never been to medical school, feeling that in order to survive financially they must squeeze in as many patients as possible, and see them in the most efficient manner, not necessarily the most beneficial.

The strains on both doctors and patients have begun to fray nerves and there is a movement underway to demand a "Patient's Bill of Rights." In the meantime it is up to you to take responsibility for your own health and well being. If you feel like your doctor isn't hearing you, or that you are unhappy with the relationship, find another doctor! One who will listen. Because it is only when we listen, that we can hear, and then heal.

I agree with Dr. Alan F. Chino, Ph.D. and Dr. Corrine D. Davis M.D. in their book ***"Validate Your Pain Exposing the Chronic Pain Cover-Up"*** (Health Access Press, 2000), "…paying attention to —and validating—the human experience of chronic pain will bring about a significant healing effect. Outcome from 'proper' physical treatment administered by an unfeeling, uncaring, dispassionate robot will be far inferior to that provided within the context of a caring, compassionate team of human beings." You hold the key to your healing. I am but a partner on the path.

I work at being an effective healer for people with pain because I myself have lived with chronic pain. I think of it as the price I paid for the many sports injuries I've suffered throughout the years.

I know what living with chronic pain can do to you, physically, emotionally and spiritually. There is a miasma of

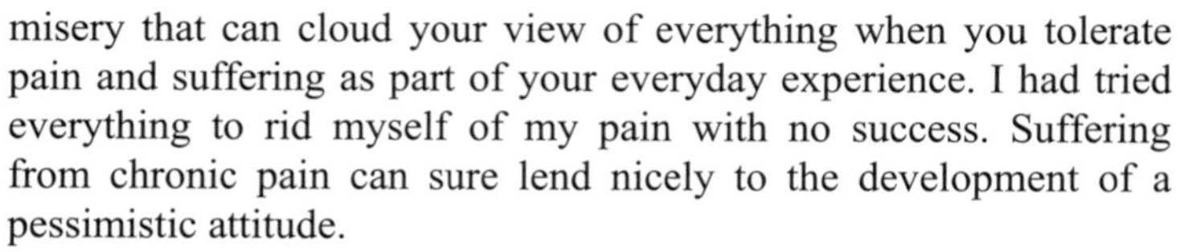

misery that can cloud your view of everything when you tolerate pain and suffering as part of your everyday experience. I had tried everything to rid myself of my pain with no success. Suffering from chronic pain can sure lend nicely to the development of a pessimistic attitude.

My closed minded misery almost cost me the opportunity to be cured. If I had not been in so much pain I doubt I would have agreed to try Prolotherapy. I mean I was a doctor and had never heard of this. But the pain was screaming, I was desperate and I put my skepticism aside. In suspending skepticism, I found relief. Miraculous relief. I found Prolotherapy and it changed my life. I had no choice but to help others the way I had been helped.

In my practice I have achieved an 85 to 90% success rate curing my patients with Prolotherapy.

I use the term Prolotherapy more than trigger point injections because as you have read, every injection of this type is really a combination of both, no matter what solution is used, or if only a needle is used without a solution.

There is a saying, "Physician heal thyself," and I do. All the chronic injuries that I sustained through my active participation in sports throughout the years have been injected (many by self-injection). This has made a dramatic change in the quality of my life.

One of the most satisfying aspects of my job is being able to prevent unnecessary surgery.

I pride myself on saving my patients from the knife. It is rare that a patient undergoes surgery after Prolotherapy. Why would anyone go under the knife and change the natural anatomy of their body by removing a part of it?

I love to take away a patient's diagnosis and educate patients that in most cases, their diagnosis is either wrong or is not

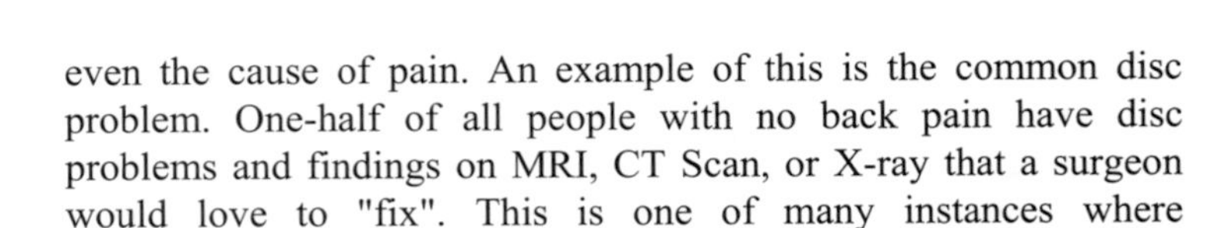

even the cause of pain. An example of this is the common disc problem. One-half of all people with no back pain have disc problems and findings on MRI, CT Scan, or X-ray that a surgeon would love to "fix". This is one of many instances where technology in diagnosis can prove harmful.

A big part of my job is opening up the doors of perception so that patients can see that they have the ability to move past the restraint of a physical diagnosis and into a place of healing. I have noticed that people who are positive in their consciousness get better faster than the others. Some people have come to identify themselves with their pain and derive purpose from it. This greatly prohibits them from healing.

I am not saying you have to love your doctor, or vice versa, but if you feel that your doctor is not responsive, not hearing you, or worse, not helping you, you owe it to yourself to find another doctor. But you must also own up to your responsibility and start the healing inside yourself. Be prepared to give up all those things that get in the way of your health. Get involved in your own recovery. Don't expect a doctor to do it for you.

Satisfaction in my work depends on patients getting better. I share my patient's highs and lows. I am as excited as they are when they start to feel better, and am as discouraged as they are if the treatment is taking longer to kick in than they had hoped. I am very involved and get very attached. I put myself in the place of the patient, which is easy to do because, after all, I have been there.

May Peace and Health Be With You,
Marc Darrow

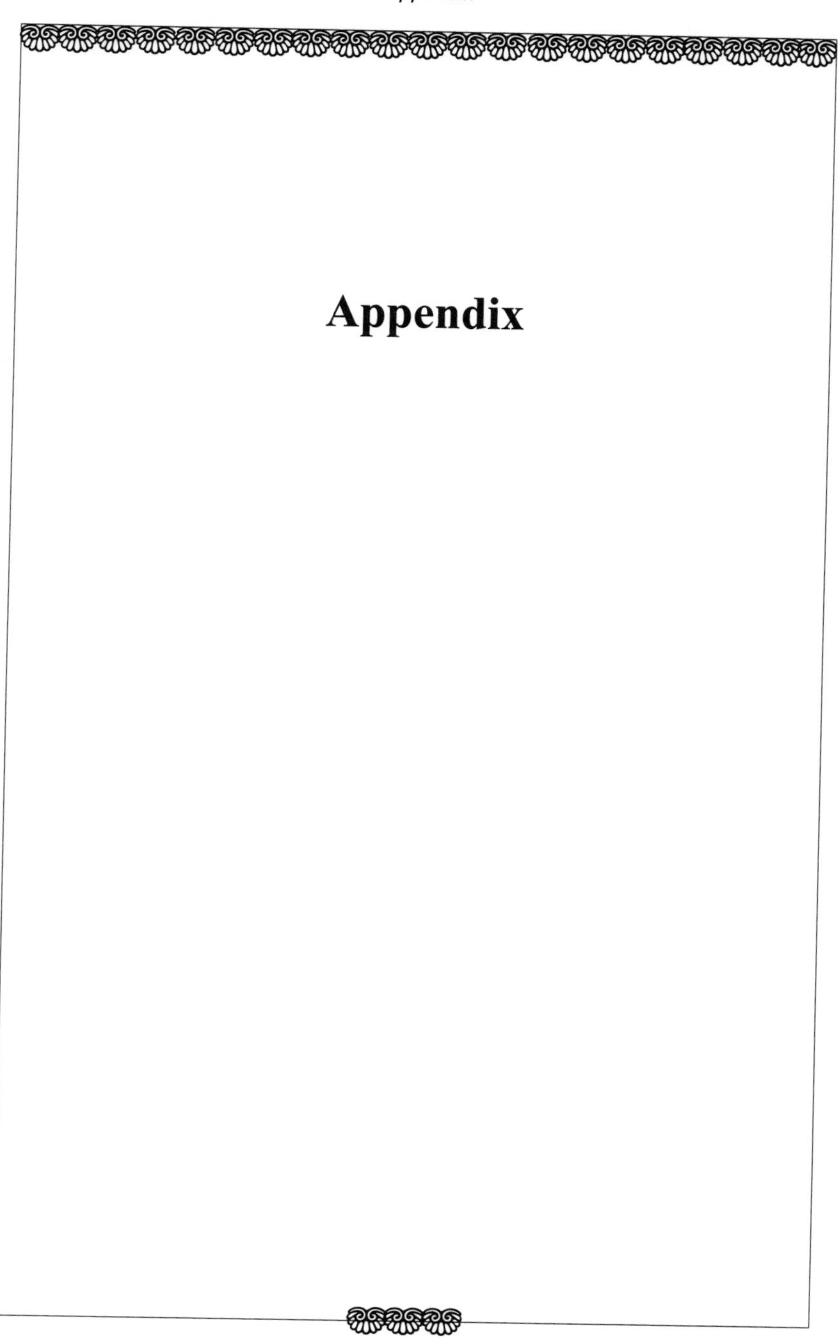

Appendix

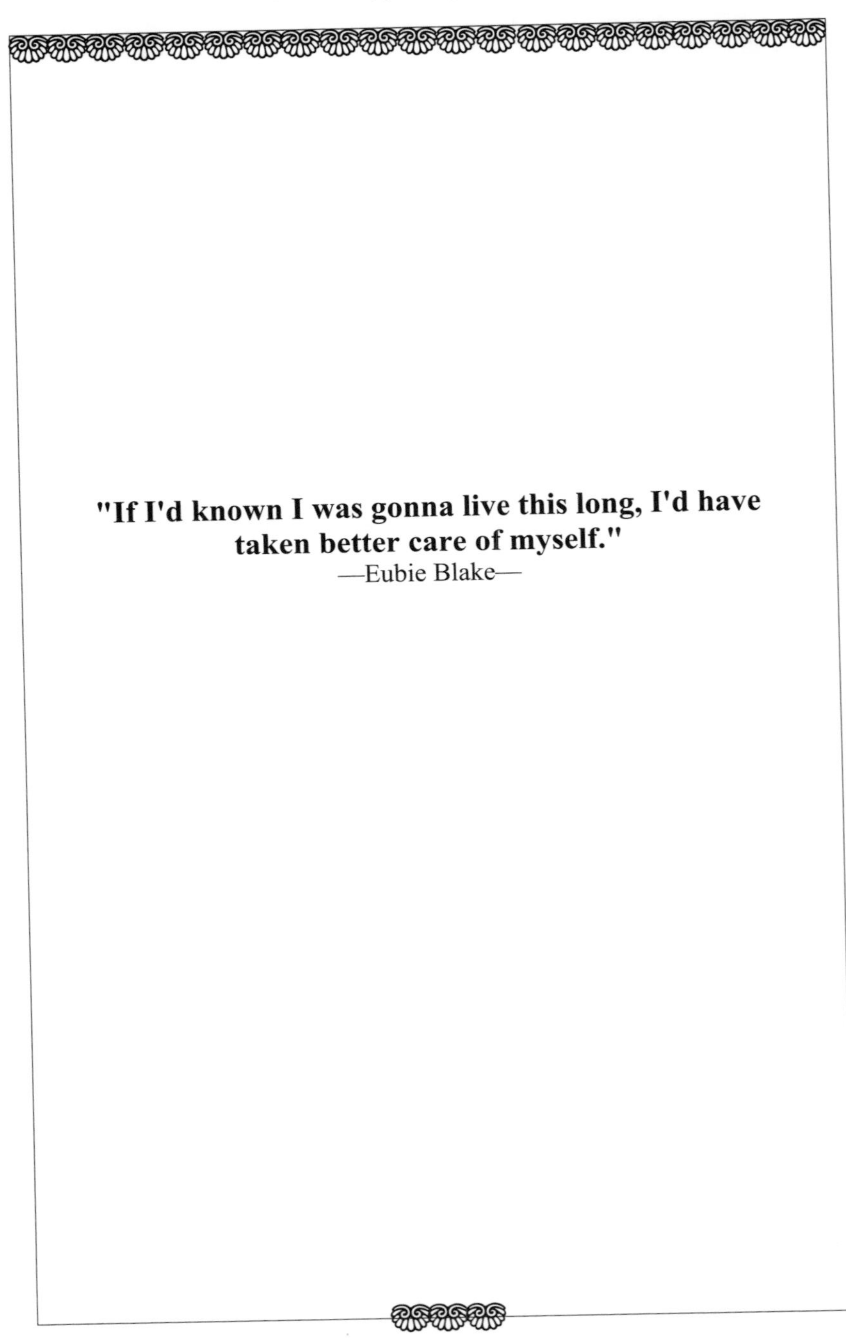

"If I'd known I was gonna live this long, I'd have taken better care of myself."

—Eubie Blake—

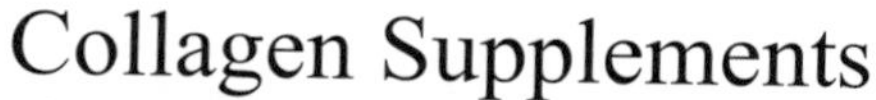

Collagen Supplements

Sarah Quadri, Bachelor of Science in Biomolecular Science

Introduction

The word "collagen" is derived from kolla, the Greek word for glue. It is the strong fiber that weaves throughout the body for strength and support to literally hold the body together like glue would. Collagen is the most abundant protein in the body with about 14 or so known types.

As we age, the body's ability to make collagen protein and its different complexes slows down. In time, a collagen deficiency occurs in the skin, joints, and other parts of the body, weakening the connective tissues that holds us together. The remaining collagen fibers may also lose their moist texture and become rigid, mainly due to free radical damage. The combined lack of collagen and dehydrated collagen can manifest itself as wrinkles; joint pain; brittle hair, skin and nails; and other connective tissue conditions.

To replace lost and replenish dried out collagen, external lotions and creams have been popular for years. Collagen injections for wrinkles are also popular. Recently, however, attention has shifted to the use of collagen as an oral supplement.

Oral supplementation of collagen provides a way in which the body can be provided vital amino acids and proteoglycans (specialized sugars in the body) important to maintenance of connective tissues. Currently, two main collagen supplements are being utilized—a combined collagen type I & collagen type III oral supplement and a collagen type II supplement, as these are the most abundant types in the body.

Collagen type I & collagen type III are the chief collagen types in hair, skin, nails, tendons, ligaments, muscles, bones, teeth, eyes, and blood vessels. Although their presence is beneficial in joint tissues, collagen type II is the true major component of joint cartilage. Collagen type II (particularly from chicken sternal cartilage) supplies vital amino acids, hyaluronic acid, chondroitin, and glucosamine for optimal articular (joint) cartilage support.

Collagen Type I & Collagen Type III

Studies have shown that more than 90% of the collagen found in the body is collagen type I & collagen type III, which are naturally found together as fibril-forming or tissue forming collagens.

The protein composition consists of nineteen amino acids responsible for growth, maintenance, and repair of the body, with unusually high proportions of the amino acids glycine and proline, as well as hydroxyproline and hydroxylysine (two amino acids unique to collagen) all found in particularly high concentration in tendons ligaments, bone, organ capsules, skin, fibrous cartilage, blood vessels and fascia.

Collagen type I provides a great deal of mechanical strength to structures like bones because of its ability to resist tension, while collagen type III is involved in the maintenance of expansile organs, wound healing, and tendon and ligament attachments.

Due to the importance of the roles of collagen type I & collagen type III, it would be logical to provide a supplement which is geared towards providing the building blocks to support collagen in the body, and this is where collagen oral supplementation fits in.

Collagen type I & collagen type III supplements can be made from bovine (beef), porcine (pork), or fish sources. When made from these sources, the product is best utilized when it is hydrolyzed, (broken down into smaller pieces on the molecular level by the addition of enzymes for better absorption.) Bovine skin offers one of the best sources of collagen type I & collagen type III with the following breakdown of amino acids*:

Alanine	8.5%	Leucine	2.9%
Arginine	7.9%	Lysine	4.2%
Aspartic Acid	5.70%	Methionine	0.78%
Cystine	0.08%	Phenylalanine	2.0%
Glutamic Acid	9.50%	Proline	13.80%
Glycine	22.80%	Serine	3.30%
Histidine	0.77%	Threonine	1.90%
Hydroxyproline	13.00%	Tyrosine	0.40%
Hydroxylysine	0.70%	Valine	2.40%
Isoleucine	1.30%		

*represent average grams amino acid per 100 grams, amounts may vary.

Note: the high levels of glycine and proline offer ideal building blocks for repair of muscles, tissues, and skin. By supplementing this natural ratio of amino acids, rather than large, random amounts of certain amino acids, an individual can receive more balanced collagen support.

Oral supplementation of collagen type I & collagen type III can be used not only for aesthetic concerns like hair, skin, and nails, but also to address damage such as a torn meniscus, back muscle problems, and even nutritional support for muscle and collagen diseases like fibromyalgia and Ehlers-Danlos syndrome.

In fibromyalgia, a disease involving unexplainable muscle pain, some speculate that some sufferers may have low amounts of collagen type III in their bodies, and this may be addressed with supplementation and nutrition. Interestingly enough, collagen type

III is especially important in that it is the earliest collagen laid down by the body in the connective tissue healing process. In the genetic disease Ehlers-Danlos syndrome, individuals lack the chromosomal marker for making collagen and suffer pain as a result. Individuals supplementing their diets with collagen type I and collagen type III have seen some relief in their symptoms, in particular when using Super Collagen™ brand of collagen type I & collagen type III (by NeoCell Corporation experienced in collagen since 1986).

Collagen Type II

Collagen type II is the major structural component of hyaline and elastic cartilage, intervertebral discs, and vitreous humour. Collagen type II, is also a fibril-forming collagen; it complexes with important carbohydrates in these areas where resistance to tension is needed.

Collagen type II extracted from chicken sternal cartilage offers the components to supply the joints with the building blocks needed for repair. The protein content of chicken collagen II is approximately 65-70% (less than collagen I & III) and 30-35% of naturally occurring mucopolysaccharides (specialized carbohydrates in the body) that includes chondroitin, glucosamine, and most importantly hyaluronic acid. The composition of chicken collagen type II protein consists of eighteen amino acids. The percentages and molecular weights are different than those found in the collagen type I & III*.

Amino acid	Amount	Amino acid	Amount
Alanine	10.79%	Lysine	4.72%
Arginine	4.81%	Methionine	1.10%
Aspartic Acid	7.95%	Phenylalanine	2.41%
Glutamic Acid	13.47%	Proline	8.75%
Glycine	24.60%	Serine	2.37%
Histidine	1.51%	Threonine	2.46%
Isoleucine	3.74%	Tyrosine	1.19%
Leucine	5.85%	Valine	4.28%

*represent average grams amino acid per 100 grams amounts may vary.

Chicken collagen type II can be unhydrolyzed, undenatured, or hydrolyzed, and there are differing views on the benefits of each. Undenatured chicken collagen type II is “native” and unprocessed, and is theorized to induce a process of oral immune tolerance to address rheumatoid arthritis. It is thought that introducing small amounts of undenatured chicken collagen to the body may trigger positive recognition of collagen type II in the body so that the body’s immune system will halt attacks of collagen type II in the joints. Small amounts are necessary because using larger amounts of native collagen type II can actually induce arthritic responses in the body.

Consistent positive results of immune application of undenatured collagen type II are still in the process in human use. It was also perceived for a period of time that like collagen type I & III, hydrolysis of chicken collagen type II would also be necessary to maximize the absorption and benefits of collagen type II as a

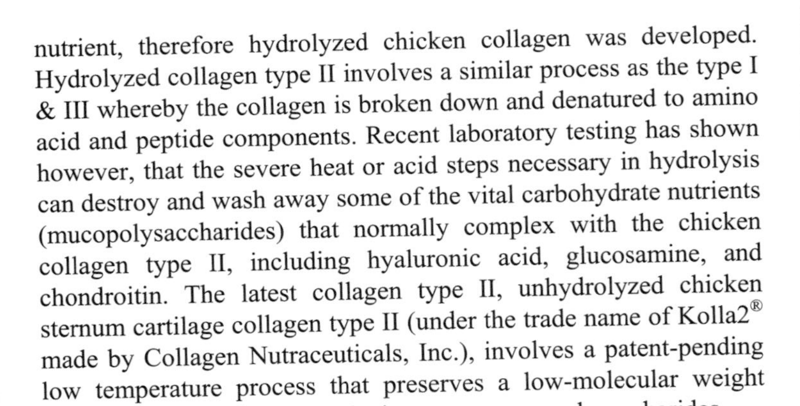

nutrient, therefore hydrolyzed chicken collagen was developed. Hydrolyzed collagen type II involves a similar process as the type I & III whereby the collagen is broken down and denatured to amino acid and peptide components. Recent laboratory testing has shown however, that the severe heat or acid steps necessary in hydrolysis can destroy and wash away some of the vital carbohydrate nutrients (mucopolysaccharides) that normally complex with the chicken collagen type II, including hyaluronic acid, glucosamine, and chondroitin. The latest collagen type II, unhydrolyzed chicken sternum cartilage collagen type II (under the trade name of Kolla2® made by Collagen Nutraceuticals, Inc.), involves a patent-pending low temperature process that preserves a low-molecular weight structure as well as more of the important mucopolysaccharides.

Researchers recognized that hydrolyzing chicken sternal collagen type II would lower the high levels of anti-inflammatory mucopolysaccharides present in the cartilage of six-week-old chicks (the source of chicken sternal collagen type II). In contrast, Kolla2® unhydrolyzed collagen type II leaves the long chains of amino acids intact, but allows the body's own superior natural enzymes to recognize the precise genetic code in the healthy active molecules of chicken sternal collagen type II for maximum assimilation. This provides chicken sternal collagen type II as a building block for the body to heal itself, especially in cases of osteoarthritis. By not hydrolyzing, the Kolla2® unhydrolyzed chicken sternal cartilage collagen type II provides the following ratio of nutrients (±2%):

50% Collagen Type II Protein
17% Hyaluronic Acid
16% Chondroitin and
about 17% Glucosamine.

The benefits of preserving the mucopolysaccharides result in the presence of the natural ratios of the building blocks the body needs to make more cartilage and other important tissues, present best in Kolla2® unhydrolyzed chicken sternal collagen type II. The

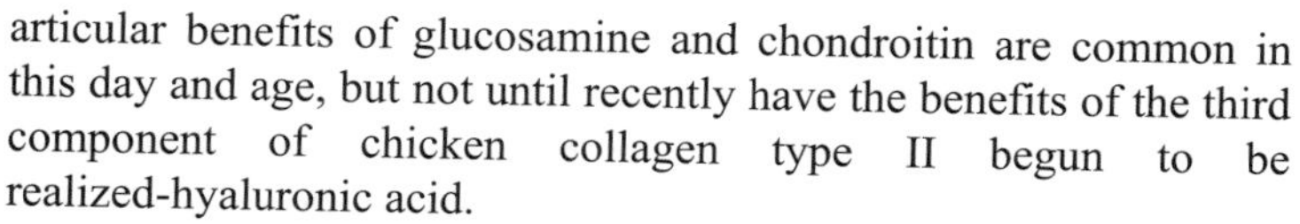

articular benefits of glucosamine and chondroitin are common in this day and age, but not until recently have the benefits of the third component of chicken collagen type II begun to be realized-hyaluronic acid.

Hyaluronic acid (HA), also known as hyaluronan, is an important disaccharide found in every tissue of the body, but in particular as an essential lubricant of healthy joints, skin and eyes. Recent attention on hyaluronic acid began after ABC News published a report on the Japanese village of Yuzuri Hara, where the residents were living long and healthy lives at much higher rates than statistics of most other peoples. After studying them, it was determined that their diets stimulated and supplied high quantities of hyaluronic acid in their bodies. In fact, to rule out the effects of genetics, younger generations of Yuzuri Hara exposed to new western foods infiltrating the region have expressed health problems and created an "upside down health pyramid" where elderly parents were outliving their adult children. Our western diets leave little room for sufficient supply of HA, therefore people have turned to the prospect of using HA-rich supplements such as PureH.A.™ natural hyaluronic acid.

HA is part of a group of macromolecules in the body labeled as glycosaminoglycans (GAGs), which are primarily in cell membranes and in the intercellular matrix of connective tissue. Along with water, HA's unique property of high viscosity, and therefore low compressibility, provides vital shock absorption and lubrication properties. In the intercellular matrix, HA essentially operates with water to "bathe" cells by binding with almost 1000-fold of its own weight in water. This distribution along with the property of high viscosity provides for separation of cells and intercellular fibers to facilitate movement of nutrients and waste, protection of underlying tissue such as cartilage, bone, and muscle from wear and tear, and hydration and structure. HA can be found more concentrated in areas of the body that endure increased movement and friction or have a higher fluid component such as the eyes, ears, heart, and joints. In the joints, HA is secreted by chondrocytes (articular cells) and is one of the most essential components of the vitreous humor (joint fluid) that protects the joints from deterioration. HA works similarly as a component of the fluids lubricating the heart to prevent friction between the heart and surrounding membranes, as well as lubrication of the corneal epithelium on the surface of the eye. HA also provides an optically clear structural component for rigidity in the vitreous (fluid) of the eye. In addition to its physical contributions, HA has also been found to assist in regulation of cell turnover in the skin, to serve as an anti-oxidant to free-radicals generated by UV radiation, and as an aid in communication between cells in cell-mediated immune response. Just as collagen, as we age HA content in our bodies tends to decrease, but recent supplementation with an HA-rich product is providing promising results.

The ability to nutritional support so many different conditions with collagen supplementation can only further interest in researching its further applications and mechanisms for support of connective tissues.

**The above statements have not been evaluated by the Food and Drug Administration. These products are not intended to diagnose, cure, or prevent any disease. Results will vary among individuals. Always consult with your physician.*

Resources and Links

48Hours.net
http://www.48hours.net
Health-related information.

ABC News - health information
http://abcnews.com

About Orthopaedics
http://orthopedics.about.com

About Sports Medicine - latest news.
http://sportsmedicine.about.com

Achoo - gateway to healthcare resources.
http://www.achoo.com/main.asp

Alternative Medicine Center
http://www.ahn.com

American Academy of Orthopaedic Surgeons Public Information
http://www.aaos.org/wordhtml/home2.htm

American Council on Science and Health
http://www.acsh.org

American Fibromyalgia Syndrome Association
http://www.afsafund.org

Body1.com
http://www.body1.com
Where technology and healthcare meet.

Centers for Disease Control and Prevention
http://www.cdc.gov

Chiropractic America
http://www.chirousa.com

ChiroWeb
http://www.chiroweb.com

CNN.com
http://www.cnn.com

Columbia University College of Physicians and Surgeons-
Complete Home Medical Guide
http://cpmcnet.columbia.edu

DiscoveryHealth.com
http://health.discovery.com

Doctor Directory
http://www.doctordirectory.com

Dr.Koop's Health Wellness Center
http://www.drkoop.com

Dr. Whitaker-Guide to Alternative Heath and Anti-Aging Medicine
http://www.drwhitaker.com

Doctors in LA
http://www.la-doctor.com/main-directory.htm"

eCureMe.com
http://www.ecureme.com

Sports eMedicine
http://www.emedicine.com

Fibromyalgia Network
http://www.fmnetnews.com

HealthAnswers
http://www.healthanswers.com

Health Care Information Resources- directory
a http://www.healthcity.com

HealthFinder
http://www.healthfinder.gov

Health Information Resources- Toll-Free Numbers for Health Information
http://www.health.gov/nhic/NHICScripts/Tollfree.cfm

Health Links Net
http://www.healthlinks.net

Health News Directory
http://www.healthnewsdirectory.com

Health News Network
http://www.healthnewsnet.com

The Health Pages
http://www.the-health-pages.com

HealthScout - daily health news and resources.
http://www.healthscout.com

HealthWeb
http://www.healthweb.org
Directory of health information.

HumanGenome Project Information
http://www.ornl.gov/hgmis

IntelliHealth
http://www.intelihealth.com
Features Harvard Medical School's Consumer Health Information.

International Society of Travel Medicine
http://www.istm.org

MDAdvice.com
http://www.mdadvice.com

MedicalProxy.com
http://www.medicalproxy.com

MedicineNet.com
http://www.medicinenet.com/Script/Main/hp.asp

MSN Health
http://health.msn.com

MSN Sports Fitness
http://content.health.msn.com

MSNBC Health News
http://www.msnbc.com/news/health_front.asp

NIH Health Information Index
http://www.nih.gov/health/InformationIndex/HealthIndex/Pubincov.htm
Health topics and government institutes providing relevant reseach - http://www.nih.gov/health/infoline.htm - toll free information lines.

People's Medical Society
http://www.peoplesmed.org/index.html

The Physician and Sports Medicine
http://www.physsportsmed.com/index.html

SpineHealth.com - Resource for back pain.
http://www.spine-health.com/index.html

Sports Medicine- links from About.com.
http://sportsmedicine.about.com

Sports Medicine
http://www.medfacts.com Sports Medicine

Sports Medicine
http://www.sportsmedicine.com

Sports Medicine
http://sportsmedicine.about.com

USAToday Health News
http://www.usatoday.com/news/health/healthindex.htm

Virtual Hospital
http://www.vh.org

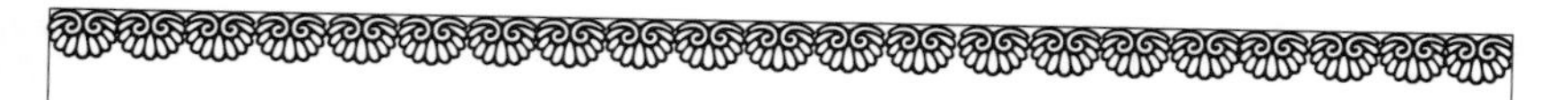

The Visible Human Project
http://www.nlm.nih.gov/research/visible/visible_human.html

WebMD
http://my.webmd.com

WholeHealthMD
http://www.wholehealthmd.com

YourSpine
http://www.yourspine.com

YourSurgery.com
http://www.yoursurgery.com/index.cfm

Prolotherapy Links

American Association of Orthopaedic Medicine
http://www.aaomed.org

American Back Institute of New Orleans on Prolotherapy
http://www.backpaininstitute.com/serv03.htm

Atkins Center for Complementary Medicine
http://atkinscenter.com

Dr.Weil on Prolotherapy
http://www.pathfinder.com/drweil/archiveqa/0,2283,1476,00.html

The Doctor's Medical Library
http://www.medical-library.net/specialties/prolotherapy.html

Evaluating Your Prolotherapist
http://www.caringmedical.com/faqtopics/prolotherapy.asp

Fact,Fiction and Fraud in Modern Medicine
http://www.dormanpub.com/home.htm

The Gale Encyclopedia of Alternative Medicine- Prolotherapy
http://www.findarticles.com/cf_dls/g2603/0006/2603000607/p1/article.jhtml

GetProlo-Prolotherapy Referral Network and newsletter.
http://www.getprolo.com

Health Plus Web: Alternative Health Directory
http://www.healthplusweb.com/alt_directory/prolotherapy.html

HealthWorldOnline
http://www.healthy.net/library/newsletters/Update/prolotherapy.htm

Online Health Analysis
http://www.digitalnaturopath.com/treat/T85137.html

ProloNews.com
http://www.prolonews.com

Prolotherapy Article
http://www.esomc.com/prolotherapy.html

Prolotherapy Article
http://www.healthplusweb.com/alt_directory/prolotherapy.html

Prolotherapy Article
http://www.correctivecare.com/pro.html

Dr. Koop's Story
http://www.wheatons.com/Prolotherapy_Endorsement_by_DrKoop.htm

Prolotherapy Article
http://www.treatingpain.com/prolothe.htm

Prolotherapy Article
http://www.drdeorio.com/prolotherapy.html

Prolotherapy.com
http://www.prolotherapy.com

Prolotherapy Article
http://www.wheatons.com/Prolotherapy.htm

Prolotherapy Article
http://www.chronicpainsolutions.com/articles/djuricsummer99.htm

Prolotherapy Article
http://www.prolodoc.com/all_about_prolotherapy.htm

Prolotherapy Article
http://treatingpain.com/prolothe.htm

Prolotherapy Articles
http://www.prolotherapy.com/documents.htm

Other Prolotherapy Physicians
Elkins Park, Pennsylvannia
Kab S. Hong, M.D.,P.C
http://www.prolotherapy-us.com

Eugene, Oregon
Eugene Sports and Orthopaedic Medcine Center
http://www.esomc.com/index.html

Federal Way, Washington
Thomas Dorman, M.D.
http://www.paracelsusclinic.com Paracelsus Clinic

Milwaukee Pain Clinic
Dr. William Faber
http://milwaukeepainclinic.com

Oak Park, IL.
Caring Medical and Rehabilitation Sports Medicine Center
http://Caringmedical.com

Santa Barbara, CA and Ashland, OR
Allen Thomashefsky, MD
http://www.drtom.net

New York, NY
Center for Sports and Osteopathic Medicine- New York
http://www.bonesdoctor.com/prolo.html

Tyler, Texas
Jim Holleman, DO
http://www.prolotherapydoc.com/index.htm

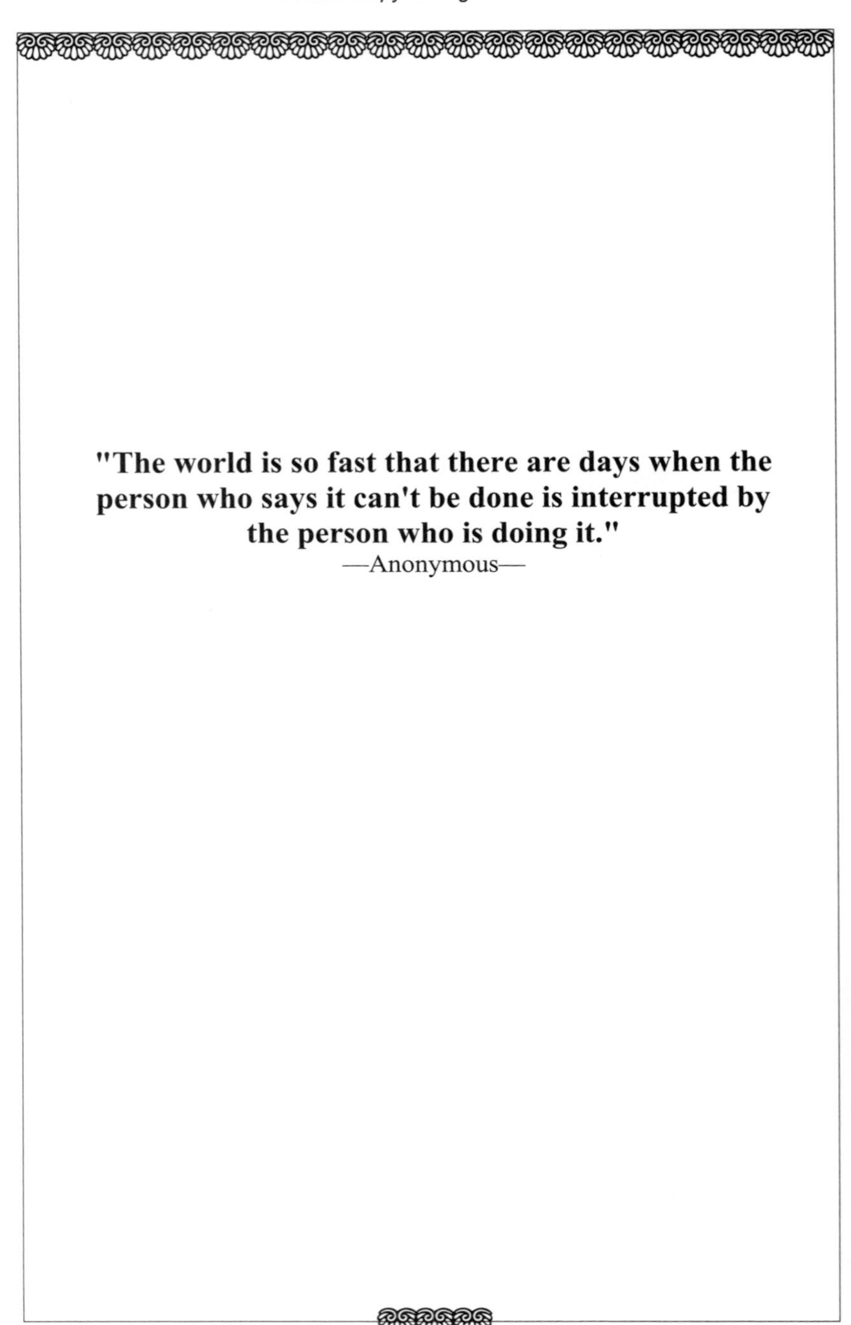
"The world is so fast that there are days when the person who says it can't be done is interrupted by the person who is doing it."
—Anonymous—

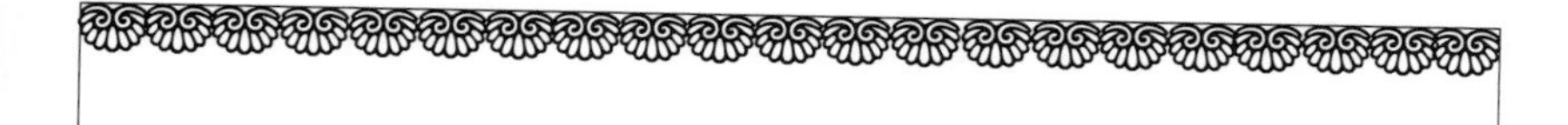

Glossary

Acupuncture
A therapy initiated in China over 5000 years ago. Much like trigger point therapy, needles are inserted into acupuncture (same points as trigger points) points to promote healing, and reduce pain. Repeated needling with acupuncture needles may proliferate collagen and promote healing much like Prolotherapy.

Acute Pain - New onset
Common kinds of acute pain are low back pain and headache which can last for several days or more. Term does not refer to the intensity of pain but the timing.

Arthritis
Breakdown of the structures in and around a joint. Bones hypertrophy as cartilage is destroyed.

Arthroscopy
A highly invasive surgical therapy which involves the use of metal scopes to diagnose damage, and drills, shavers and other tools to cut and remove tissue and bone from the joints.

Articular cartilage
The glassy cartilage covering the ends of bones. Without it bones grind and cause pain.

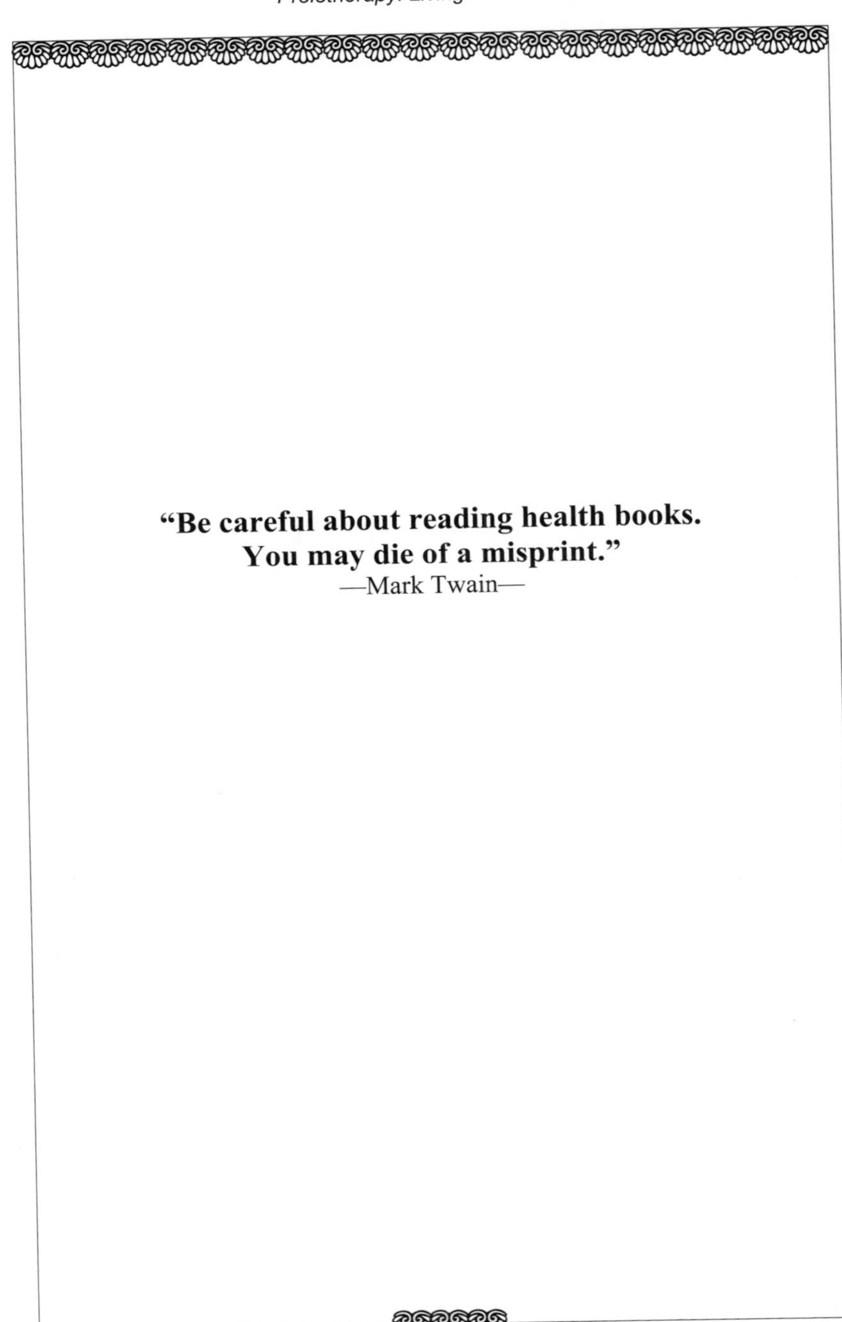

**"Be careful about reading health books.
You may die of a misprint."**
—Mark Twain—

Avascular
An area of the body such as cartilage that is not fed well by blood. Vascular refers to vessels.

Bursa
Sacs of fluid that protect tendons, muscles and ligaments from rubbing on bone.

Bursitis
Refers to inflammation of the term it follows. In this case inflammation of the bursa.

Carpal tunnel syndrome (CTS)
An impingement of the median nerve at the wrist often caused by repetitive motion.

Cartilage
Connective tissue made out of collagen. Found in the joints and covering bone where it acts as a smooth surface for gliding. See also Articular cartilage.

Chiropractic
Hands on therapy that balances the body. Newer forms of chiropractic such as AK (Applied Kinesiology) relieve pain and promote mobility and healing without forced adjustments.

Chondroitin sulfate
A nutritional supplement that is a building block of cartilage.

Chondromalacia patellae
Breaking down of the cartilage on the back of the knee bone. A type of arthritis.

Chronic Pain
Pain generally lasting more than 3 months. Patients are often disabled by their pain and may suffer severe depression and anxiety, and drug abuse.

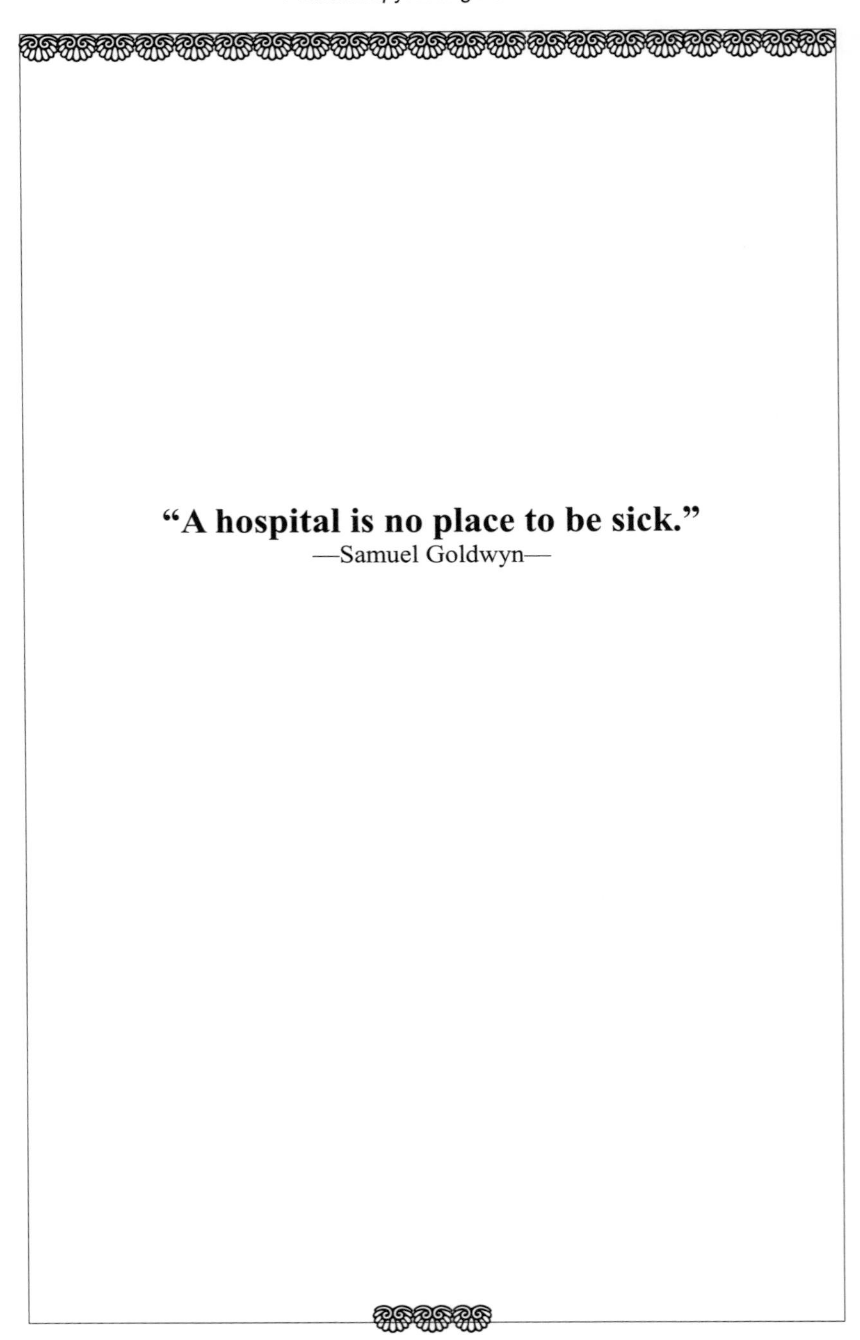

"A hospital is no place to be sick."
—Samuel Goldwyn—

Collagen
A major structural protein, the glue that holds our bodies together. Collagen is formed with molecular cables that strengthen the tendons and vast, resilient sheets that support the skin and internal organs.

Connective tissues
The soft-non-bone tissues in the body that hold us together. Examples are ligaments, muscle fascia, joint capsules and tendons.

Corticosteroids
Anti-inflammatory steroids, often injected, which reduce inflammation and pain but in doing so, interfere with the body's natural healing cascade. An example is cortisone.

Etiology
The cause of a disease or pathology.

Fascia
The connective tissue that envelops the muscles and provides support and attachment to the bones.

Fibroblasts
Cells that produce collagen.

Fibromyalgia
A complicated syndrome involving wide spread pain and fatigue, often with insomnia. It is a wastebasket diagnosis for unsolved reasons for pain.

Glucosamine sulfate
A nutritional supplement that acts to reduce joint pain. It is a building block of cartilage.

Inflammation or healing cascade
The body's natural response to injuries. It begins with inflammation (swelling and pain), which triggers an influx of fibroblasts that produce collagen and rejuvenate the tissue.

"The only thing wrong with immortality is that it tends to go on forever."
—Herb Caen—

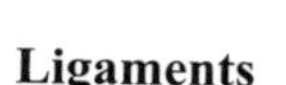

Ligaments
Strong elastic bands of connective tissue that connect bone to bone at the joints of the body.

Meniscus
A cushion in the knee joint made out of collagen.

Muscle
Contractile tissue that flexes and stretches, giving movement to the various parts of the musculoskeletal structure.

Musculoskeletal
Relating to the framework of the body composed of bones that are connected and supported by muscle and other soft tissue.

Myofascial
Relating to a type of pain in the network of connective soft tissue that covers the muscular system.

NSAIDs
All prescription and non-prescription anti-inflammatory drugs not containing steroids are classified as "non-steroidal anti-inflammatory drugs" or "NSAIDs." Examples of NSAIDs are ibuprofen, Motrin, aspirin, Naprosyn, Dapro, Celebrex, Vioxx, and an endless multitude of others. Their side effects include gastrointestinal bleeding with occasional death, and kidney and liver problems.

Patellofemoral syndrome
Painful knee condition occurring from mistracking of the patella in the femur (thigh bone). Common in runners.

Physiatrist
A medical doctor who has a specialty in Physical Medicine and Rehabilitation.

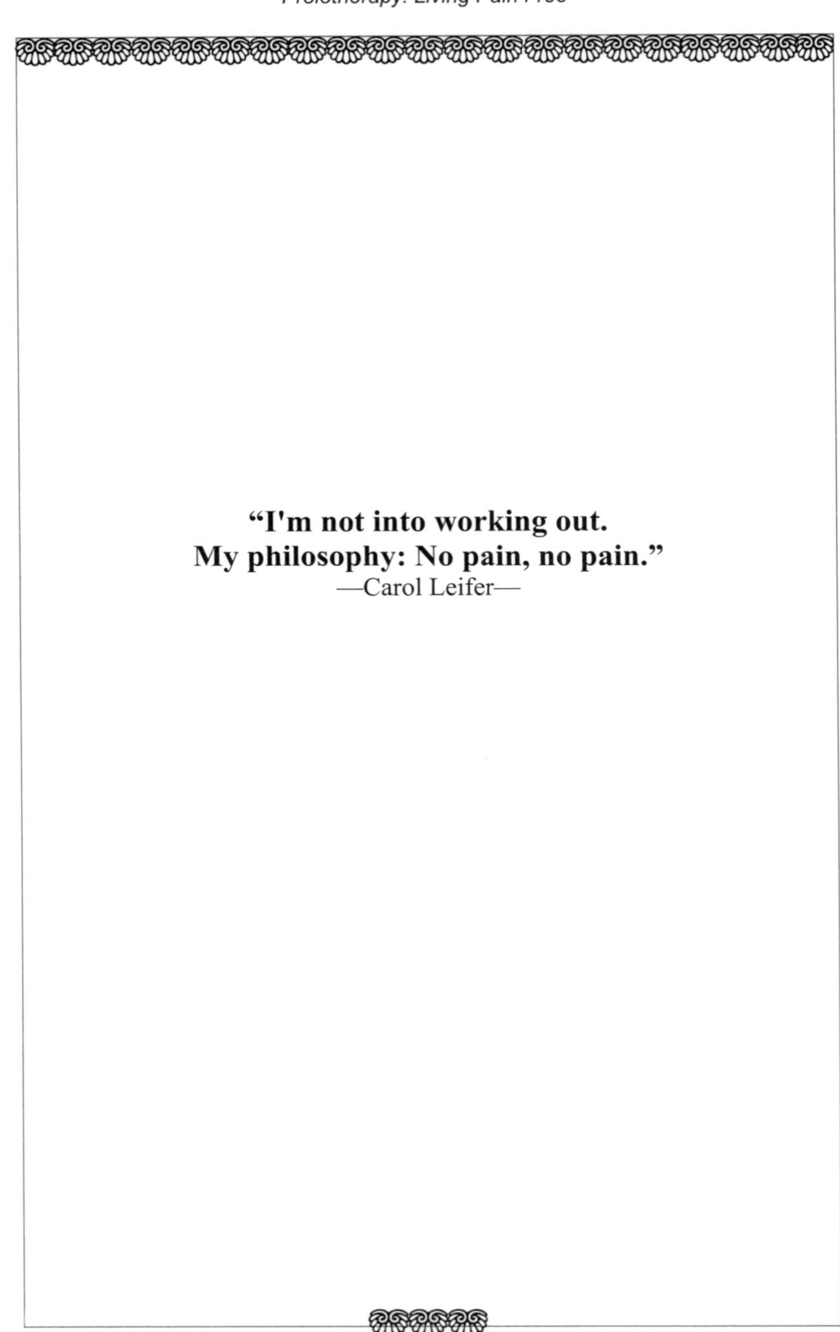

“I'm not into working out.
My philosophy: No pain, no pain.”
—Carol Leifer—

Prolotherapy
Natural simulation of the body to produce or proliferate collagen. The process rejuvenates the musculoskeletal system and reduces or eliminates pain.

Referred Pain
Pain manifested in distant areas away from the active trigger point.

RICE protocol
A treatment in which Rest, Ice, Compression, and Elevation are used after injury to prevent inflammation.

Tendinitis/Tendonitis
Inflammation of a tendon.

Tendons
Sheets of collagen that connect muscle to bone.

Trigger points
According to Janet Travel, MD, taut, tender tissue in muscles that refer pain and create dysfunction. They are the same points as acupuncture points. Muscles, tendons, ligaments and joints may have trigger points.

Trigger point injection
Injections that reduce pain in trigger or tender point areas. Trigger point injections may also proliferate collagen secondary to the inflammation caused by needle trauma, and in effect be Prolotherapy. Janet Travel, M.D. who popularized trigger point therapy, mentions in her book that a patient may be sore for a day or so after injections. It is obvious that this discomfort is a result of needle induced inflammation.

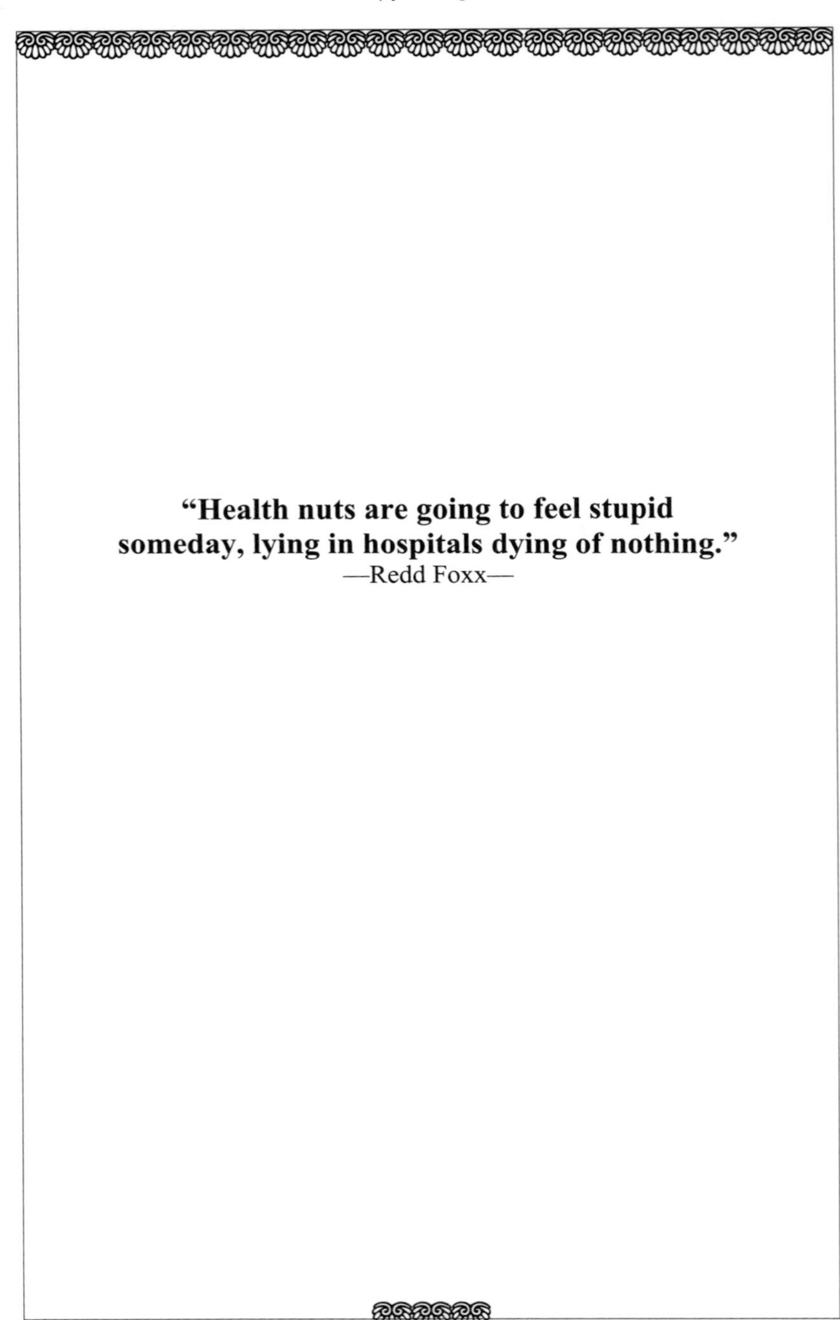

"Health nuts are going to feel stupid someday, lying in hospitals dying of nothing."

—Redd Foxx—

INDEX

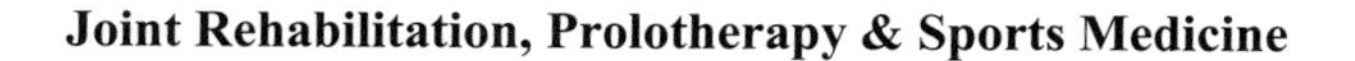

Joint Rehabilitation, Prolotherapy & Sports Medicine

A Holistic Center
For Professional and Amateur Athletes

We are a holistic center for education and prevention programs, non surgical treatments and rehabilitation for professional and amateur athletes, including weekend warriors and adventurists, designed to eliminate acute or chronic pain due to sports injuries.

Our multidisciplinary staff, all athletes themselves, work as a team with each athlete to develop a personalized program to return the person to his or her normal activities as quickly as possible, to prevent future injuries, and maintain a peak level of fitness.

Pain may result from medical disorders, such as: carpal tunnel syndrome, fibromyalgia, chronic fatigue syndrome, TMJ, arthritis, neuromuscular degeneration, or spinal stenosis, as well as from automobile accidents and sports related injuries, including those that occurred many years ago.

If you participate in any kind of sport, you are likely to incur injuries that may appear to heal, but 5, 10 or 20 years later may come back as pain of unknown origin. If you work at a repetitive task, you may not notice that you are injuring yourself at first, but over time can lead to severe pain, such as carpal tunnel syndrome and other repetitive stress injuries.

An evaluation can help pinpoint these areas and a treatment plan will help prevent the injury from becoming a permanent or recurring problem.

Joint Rehabilitation, Prolotherapy & Sports Medicine

Pain is Not Just Physical

Our philosophy on healthcare is to assist our patients in their healing process on many levels beyond just the physical.

Although our training teaches us to focus on the physical body as the cause of pain and disease, we have found that many of our physical problems stem from and are modulated by emotional, mental, psychological, and spiritual issues.

Not all people heal on the same schedule or in the same way. We provide a healing model with a loving environment. We don't deal in disease; we deal in healing, which is an active process. Our patients are taught to create the concept and feeling of health. We often have to remove a person's diagnosis that he or she has been branded with by other doctors.

Pain does not mean that a person is broken. X-rays and MRI scans frequently do not tell the truth. A common response from patients is "I can't believe this is a medical office. You are all so understanding and supportive." Many of our patients have been to a multitude of other doctors. We need to be different to make the difference.

Our support staff is the heartbeat of our philosophy. We are ever ready to assist you with scheduling, insurance filing and answering your questions.

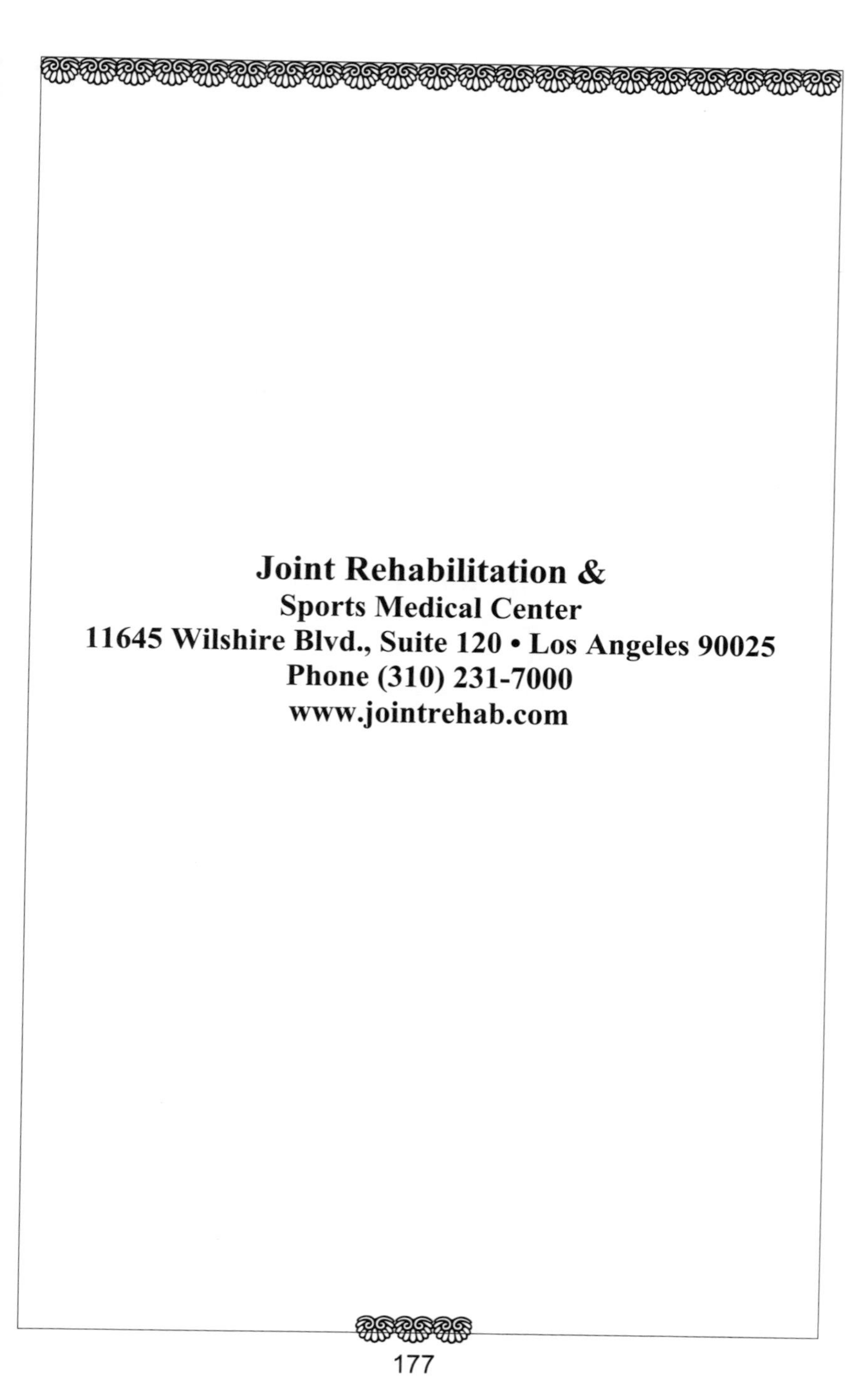
Joint Rehabilitation &
Sports Medical Center
11645 Wilshire Blvd., Suite 120 • Los Angeles 90025
Phone (310) 231-7000
www.jointrehab.com

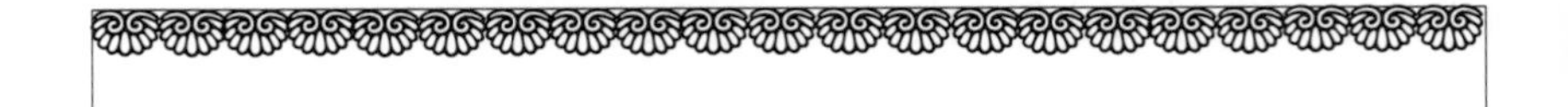

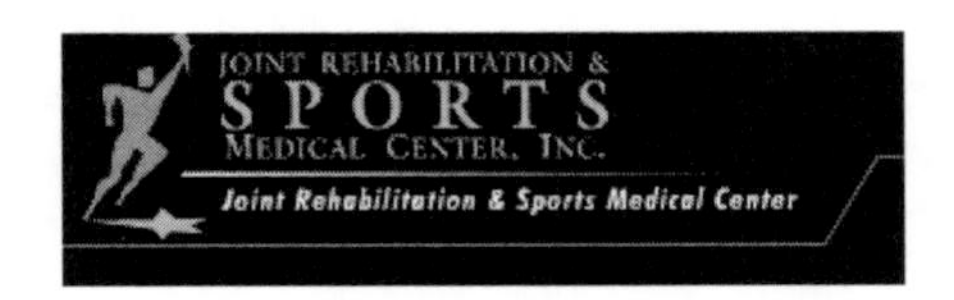

www.jointrehab.com

Keep in touch....
sign up for our free weekly e-newsletter.

Every week you can read about people and treatments for chronic pain management. Newsletters cover many topics including headaches, neck pain, shoulder pain, back pain elbow, pain, wrist pain, hip pain, knee pain, ankle pain, and foot pain.

Visit our site and sign-up!

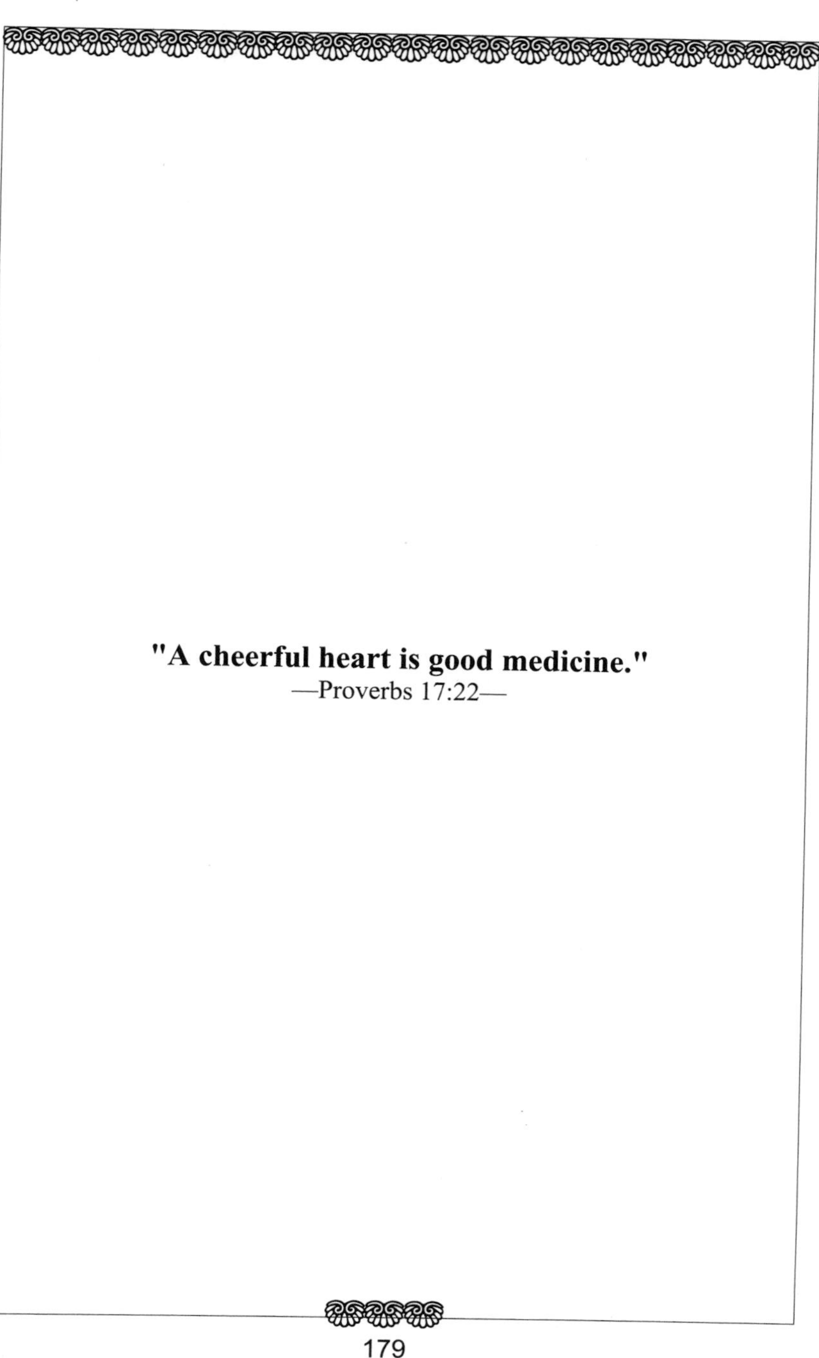

"A cheerful heart is good medicine."
—Proverbs 17:22—

About the Author

Dr. Marc Darrow is a Board Certified Physiatrist specializing in Physical Medicine and Rehabilitation. He is also an Assistant Clinical Professor at the University of California at Los Angeles's, School of Medicine.

As medical director of the Joint Rehabilitation & Sports Medicine Center in Los Angeles, Dr. Darrow has focused his practice on musculoskeletal injury, pain management, electro-diagnosis (EMG/NCS), and sports medicine and rehabilitation.

Along with Jason Kelberman, D.C., the Director of Chiropractic Services and Bill Bergman, Ph.D., director of the MedX Department, and their staff, they bring healing to patients who have searched far and wide for the answer to their health.

The approach Dr. Darrow uses is threefold. He calls it the *Trinity of Healing*, and focuses equally on all three aspects.

1. **Treat the physical body that needs the repair,**

2. **Address the mind that lives in that body and deals with the pain, and;**

3. **Attempt to move the patient's focus to the spiritual value of his or her experience. In essence to transcend the physical and move to a higher consciousness.**